THE ULTIMATE NUTRITION

Your perfect guide to optimised nutrition for a healthy lifestyle

THE ULTIMATE NUTRITION

Your perfect guide to optimised nutrition for a healthy lifestyle

Nash Jocic

Ultimate Shape Limited

London 2009

This edition published 2009 in Great Britain by
Ultimate Shape Limited
PO BOX 497 48
London
N20 0SJ

A catalogue record for this book is available from the British Library.

FIRST EDITION

Published in United Kingdom

ISBN 978-0-9562598-0-6

To my wife Victoria and children Nicol and Milos
with love and appreciation

Contents

Preface

Science has been divided about the issue of nutrition ever since modern research started fuelling so many different nutritional theories. In order to gain enough credibility, nutritional theories have required scientific research to support their conclusions. Interestingly enough, while science should have been neutral in this process (i.e. objective analysis of the different issues that come from the world around us), when it comes to the subject of nutrition, we have ended up with very different, and often contradictory, conclusions!

Scientific research has advanced at great speed, bringing many "fundamental" conclusions regarding the perfect way to eat in order to achieve better health and an improved quality of life. The problem is that, increasingly, we have been confronted with more and more conclusions and nutritional advice, all completely different, and all apparently backed up by carefully implemented scientific research! Unfortunately, it has become very clear that, depending on which camp the scientific research originates from, the answers can be predicted even before the final results and conclusions of the research have been reached.

At a basic level, the world of nutritional education has been split between the meat-diet and vegetarian-diet advocates. Consequently, in the case of meat-dominant diets, researchers can be expected to conclude that meat is the best food for us and should be the staple component of any diet. Naturally, these researchers generally always arrive at this meat-friendly conclusion. In the vegetarian diet scenarios, researchers usually conclude that plant foods are our best option, in that they will offer us the best health and longest life.

As you can imagine, given these contradictory viewpoints, the general public has become confused about nutrition. What else would one expect confronted with two completely opposite viewpoints, both "backed" by science? Either it's the total absence of meat in vegetarian diets, or the complete absence of fruits and most vegetables in diets that predominantly advocate meat and fat content as the healthiest solution.

The more "eclectic" nutrition experts often cite a "perfect" diet as containing a balance of all food groups, criticising any option which might exclude a major food group. Sounds great at first, but which major food groups do they select? They would start with vegetables, fruits, then grains, followed by meat and milk products. They simply add to the "choice" of food groups everything that is on the table, whatever people are eating, whether it is healthy or not! I totally disagree with this approach. Grains and milk products simply cannot be categorized with food groups such as vegetables, fruits and meat. The very simple reason for this is that grains and milk products didn't exist for 99% of our human evolution. These food products only appeared within the human diet some 10,000 years ago and since then we have developed all of the chronic diseases that are devastating the human species. Cancer, diabetes, cardiovascular diseases, allergies, obesity, bone deformities and tooth decay were almost unknown to our ancestors, who relied exclusively on meat, vegetables and fruit in their diets. Can this fact be any more telling? And can we, the people of the 21st century, be any more ignorant? Well, the fact that we ignore thousands of years of human dietary history doesn't help much. Yet here we are now, the only species on the planet that can travel into space and create art, literature and science, but can't work out the best and healthiest type of food to eat and in what combination.

Because of all this great confusion about nutrition, I have decided to get involved and help people to live more healthily and look better, lose body fat and increase energy levels and strength. One would need a lot of courage to tackle the misinformation, don't you agree? I understood from the very beginning that, in order to succeed, my advice and teaching in the fields of health and nutrition have to be built on the basis of my own experience. I could have advised just on the basis of morality or good character, but I simply couldn't give advice on anything that hadn't given me or my clients successful results in the first place. Once I had personally witnessed astonishing results in fat loss and strength gain, both in myself and with all my existing clients, through my particular approach to nutrition and to exercise, training systems and techniques, I was ready to offer my experience to the general public.

While most nutritional theories were, and still are, based on scientific research on animals and controlled groups of people (usually people in hospitals and with varying health conditions), I have had to deal with real, healthy people (and never experimental animals). I have also had to deliver them a promise: to help them lose extra body fat, increase their strength and lean muscle tissue, and to enjoy the benefits of improved health. My knowledge and understanding of nutrition and physical exercise doesn't come only from theoretical knowledge (as is the case with most of the nutritional and exercise "experts"). I have had to fight my own battles first, achieve results in the gym and with my own diet, and then report back about my own hard learned lessons.

After winning many wars against inactivity, obesity, malnutrition, and unhealthy lifestyles in case after case (with many, many clients), I have decided to offer my experience and knowledge to anyone who is interested in being healthier and looking better. In short, my practice hasn't been decided by biased theories; my theories have been born from my own practical engagement in the field of nutrition and weight training and through the overwhelming results that have come out of it.

My own experience was not much different to that of millions of other people who have decided to take charge of their health, strength, appearance and life in general. I started out like this: once I had decided to learn more about nutrition, I began to buy books about eating healthily. Following their advice, I ended up eating mainly grains, some vegetables and a bit of fruit with moderate or limited amounts of meat, chicken and fish.

I do have to admit that the diet tasted great and I was always looking forward to the next meal; however, the only "little" problem that had developed after 10 months of following that diet was that I ended up going from 87 kg to 115 kg in body weight, with most of the gain being from body fat!

Once I realised that all that grain indulgence would get me nowhere, the next option was a diet high in protein and fat but without fruits, vegetables and grains. I tried it, but after losing 20 kilograms in 4 months, I felt weak, tired and far from being in great shape or condition. I had lost weight, but I didn't lose as much fat as I expected. Obviously weight loss in this case didn't have much to do with fat loss. That was my first lesson about fat loss and its relation to weight loss. And that was a very expensive lesson indeed!

Just try to imagine how a young guy would feel after a huge fat gain, followed by a massive weight loss (mainly muscle mass) even though he was trying to follow all the "right" advice in order to achieve the best possible results. Staying motivated and still managing to find some will power to continue and do better after following so many wrong tracks was an arduous and often frustrating task (especially as I had only followed the best information that was available to me at the time).

However, you don't have to make the same mistakes I made. Using my experience which I share with you in this book will save you a great deal of time, money, and frustration, and will also help you to stay motivated and maintain consistency in achieving the great results that are within your reach.

After trying out so many different nutritional theories, I had no other options left but to try something that nobody else had advocated, something that was very different from the mainstream thinking about nutrition. I needed a diet that was going to be neither high in carbohydrates, nor based mainly on meat. I started experimenting with food that would not make me bloated and cause water retention, but at the same time would not make me feel sick and weak all the time. This had to be a diet that was not only based on high quantities of meat, chicken, fish and eggs – which I had tried but didn't like much – but also a diet that was not based on loads of rice, potatoes, porridge and other starches that are considered "energy giving" foods. Previously, I had religiously followed a carbohydrate-heavy diet as well, and apart from bloating, water retention, high blood-pressure and more body fat than I had ever had before, I didn't achieve much more success in terms of my physical appearance and health. In the end, I realized that both of these heavily promoted popular diets that I had experimented with for years had to be discarded in favour of a new nutritional approach, a type of diet that no one else was advocating.

My decision was to try a diet that would give me enough protein to support my muscle growth through intensive weight training, and yet enough vegetables to help me to digest and better absorb the protein while also adding extra minerals, vitamins and enzymes. Fat was to be included in controlled amounts through fish oil, olive oil and a bit of fat from eggs and red meat. Fruit was also allowed for the purposes of energy, fibre, enzymes and the micro-elements necessary for food metabolism, but not in huge amounts.

After months of experimenting with different foods and new combinations of foods, I finally came up with a nutritional solution that offered me a lot of energy, new muscle growth and a constant feeling of well-being, satisfaction and completeness. I also lost all those food cravings that are so common with protein-only diets and diets overly high in carbohydrates.

During the time I was developing my new diet, I felt like I was discovering a new continent! But despite my great personal changes and improvements, I couldn't gain approval and acceptance from people involved in the same business as me, people who were constantly trying to improve in sports and business. The new type of diet I had discovered and proved to be successful wasn't in accordance with mainstream thinking and wasn't supported by mainstream nutritional authorities. Because I was going against conventional wisdom, I didn't gain many "friends" along the way.

During this time I started to do a lot of personal training, strength coaching, and life coaching, and I was fully dedicated to changing people's lives (at least those who approached me) to help them lose fat, get stronger, look better and feel much better about themselves in general. Using time-tested training techniques and my new nutritional approach, I started achieving wonders with my clients! One after another they started getting in shape, losing body fat, becoming stronger and improving their self-confidence as they never had before. Good news spread like wildfire and very quickly I had so many people who wanted to start training with me that I couldn't take them all on. It was then I realised that, in order to help more people to get in shape and live more healthily, I would have to start delivering my information in a way that could reach a wider audience. The first thought that came to my mind was to write a book about nutrition that would finally help people understand the fundamentals of healthy eating and provide a diet that everyone could follow successfully in order to lose fat, stay healthy and improve their quality of life.

In late 1988 I published my first book about nutrition entitled "Body-building Nutrition". It was another 20 years before I sat down in front of my laptop again to try to give the public an insight into the way of eating that I have found absolutely perfect in achieving and maintaining perfect health, great shape and an optimal level of mental and physical strength; the way of eating that has helped me to get in shape and stay in the same great shape for the last 25 years; the way of eating which has been followed by thousands of my clients that I have personally supervised and trained, or advised and guided worldwide with outstanding success. The understanding and guidance that you will gain from this book about how food relates to human evolution, and the ultimate health and strength that every one of us is entitled to, comes from my life-long passion and determination to help people achieve a high quality of life through healthy eating, effective exercise and a lifestyle that everyone deserves.

This book would never have been written if I hadn't personally witnessed the positive results that my clients have achieved throughout all these years. Their results were my biggest inspiration and encouragement to continue what I had started doing in the early eighties. The satisfaction that I have enjoyed every time a client loses an extra pound of body fat or lifts a few more pounds while doing a bench press or biceps curl has been overwhelming. The satisfaction of seeing incredible changes in one person's life when they lost the 50 or 60 pounds of extra body fat they had carried for more than 40 years, or someone who was skinny all their life weighing around 150 pounds with 20% of body fat, now standing in front of me weighing 200 pounds with only 7% body fat! Achieving results like these have sometimes made me feel like I have been blessed...

This is the first time, my dear friend, that you will have an opportunity to read a book written by someone who was on the front line (as I like to say) and still is. I'm still training daily with great passion and great intensity, still training people and advising clients from all around the world, achieving positive results with all of them without a single failure through a proven routine that works in 100% of cases. Today, I'm still eating the same food and following the same diet that you will find in this book and that after all these years continues to deliver great results!

The content of this book should be understood as the result of my own experience and the experience of thousands of people that I have personally supervised through personal consulting, online life coaching and personal training, nutritional advice and strength coaching in various different forms. My personal involvement in tailoring the individual programs and advice has to be taken into consideration when applying the content of this book to your own nutritional program and lifestyle strategy.

Despite my utmost efforts to make this book helpful to everyone who reads it, individual differences have to be taken into account when implementing some or all of the nutritional approaches suggested in this book.

Before starting any nutritional or exercise program, consult your physician and make sure that you are in good enough health to allow you to implement these new changes. The nutritional advice that you will find in this book will always work much better if it is associated with regular and effective exercise as a part of a healthy lifestyle.

Introduction

There has been so much said and so many books written about food, nutrition, proper diet, detoxification, correct calorific intake etc., that it is very hard to imagine that there are any people left who don't really understand nutrition. After everything that has been offered to the public through books and the media to improve our knowledge of nutrition, how can there be any individuals or larger groups of people left that have not gotten these messages on nutrition and implemented them into their daily lives and everyday habits?

Let's look at the reality though, at the everyday world for the majority of people out there today. Chronic diseases, the ones that can be attributed directly to our eating habits, are constantly on the rise, yet cosmetic changes to our bodies are ringing the alarm bells the loudest. We are all getting fatter! And once we become bigger we need to eat more, so we become bigger consumers who need to spend more on food, whilst our health expenses also continue to rise. Once we get diagnosed as a sufferer of chronic disease we also instantly become a lifetime customer of the pharmaceutical industry. It's a never-ending cycle.

Everything could be alright if this irresponsible behaviour didn't cost as much as it does. Billions are spent every year in order to cure, compensate for and correct diseases which can be prevented with a more responsible eating approach and more sensitive eating habits. Almost all chronic diseases are exacerbated or caused by improper nutrition – either the wrong selection of food or simply over-eating (and in some cases under-eating). In this day and age when we know more about nutrition than ever before, and when we should also be benefitting health-wise more than ever, we are actually suffering more diet-related health problems than at any point in our human history!

People were often much healthier in the days when the science of nutrition didn't even exist, without knowing about all the food components, theories of food combining, calorie counting and the other great discoveries in the field of nutrition that we are so proud of today. So the question that ultimately arises is what could our ancestors possibly have done right that we are consistently doing wrong?

In order to understand the reasons for the absence of modern day chronic diseases before the advent of our present day society, we need to analyse our ancestors' lifestyle. We need to look at their food choices and food availability, as well as other factors that have directly influenced the physiological development of our species.

My intention has never been to underestimate the powerful factors in our modern lives that are driving us towards a poor diet, overeating, starvation or other physical stresses such as depression, emptiness, boredom, insecurity etc.; it has been to underline the most important factor of them all, which is the information that is made available to us. Only the correct information can stimulate and lead to the right course of action. In my long experience, working with thousands of people around the globe, I have come to the conclusion that everyone reacts positively and creatively once presented with the right information! Results may vary depending on other factors, but motivation, consistency and determination can only begin with the presentation of the right information and proper guidelines.

In the attempt to find the most perfect diet that will enable us to function optimally with perfect health, we have to get away from different dogmas directly related to nutrition. Religion, culture, family tradition, social trends and similar extremely powerful factors usually contribute to the formation of one's dietary choices. This is the main reason why we have such a huge diversity when it comes to different diets and eating habits around the world. Not surprisingly, people always believe that the "traditional" ways of eating are the healthiest and best ways. I have heard so many different stories from different corners of the world, and always with the same aim – to convince me that a particular diet from a particular place is the most perfect, healthy diet guaranteeing a great looking physique!

Well, it may sound interesting the first time, but after hearing the same story over and over again, regardless of which part of the world it originates from, you have to ask yourself, can it be true? Even completely opposing diets promise the same results: good health and a great physical appearance!

In order to sever this Gordian knot we have to look back into the human evolutionary cycle and try to understand how we (Homo sapiens) have evolved, taking into account the kinds of food that we have developed around. This will point us in the right direction to answer questions concerning the compatibility of the human digestive system with the food that we eat regularly nowadays.

Human physiology is the same for all humans, regardless of race, religion, nationality or culture, and therefore we all generally respond the same to the same food. Our biochemistry responds the same to stimuli such as the food that we ingest. Once food enters the digestive system and starts getting broken down, our internal sensors start recognizing the different macro- and micronutrients and our system responds by secreting different enzymes, hormones and other chemicals in order to make the most from the life supporting components that have been introduced. We can have different tolerances to different particular food components, such as lactose, fibre etc, and we can also have allergic reactions to different foods, but generally we all respond the same regarding the basic macronutrients.

Our physiological response is generally also the same regarding different medications. This is why millions of us (with some exceptions) get treated with the same medications (penicillin, etc.) after being infected with the same bacteria or virus. So, why would we respond differently to the same food? The fact is: we do not. And because we do respond the same to the same food, there isn't much to support the argument that different diets will produce the same exact results.

Humans are capable of eating different foods and surviving on them even though these foods may not be the healthiest and best for us. But in this book we are not talking about surviving; we are talking about finding the healthiest and most advantageous food that will help us optimise our unique human potentials. There is only one type of diet, the only right selection of different foods that will benefit us all, regardless of any differences that we have mentioned.

Food: Where it All Begins

The existence of life, from each individual cell to the whole organism, is not possible without a constant supply of nutrients. Amino acids, essential fats, glucose, water and a whole spectrum of enzymes and micronutrients are necessary compounds that enable the continuation of life in its various forms. Without these essential elements, no cell or organism can exist. These life-supporting components are all obtained by the body through the food that we eat.

The food that nature has created and made available to every different species is perfectly tailored to support life and continued health. Every single species grows and lives around particular types of foods which are compatible with their physiology. Those foods give them the opportunity to optimise their genetic potential, and improve their chances for survival through natural selection. During famines, we witness many cases of individual starvation within species, and sometimes starvation of the entire species, which is actually caused by a lack of suitable foods. Although other foods may be available, they aren't eaten. Many species would rather starve themselves instead of eating food that is not meant for them! Why? Commanded by instincts (unconscious behavioural patterns inherited through generations with the single goal of self-protection), non-human species avoid any foods that pose a serious threat to their health. Although we may classify species that can eat anything in order to survive as being more adaptable with a better chance of survival, that may not necessarily be an advantage from nature's point of view. As we humans know very well, illness and poor health can be passed on to successive generations, thereby creating deadly chronic diseases. Interestingly enough, no species other than humans suffers from chronic diseases! What do humans eat?

Our ability to eat just about any kind of food has helped us to survive and overcome the times when some types of foods were not available, such as during periods of drought, famine and floods, through the ice ages, during extinction of other species, etc. But our ability to thrive on any type of food developed into bad habits when, even in situations where healthy and beneficial foods were abundant, we carried on eating foods that had unhealthy consequences. We can eat grains, vegetables, fruit, nuts, roots, meats, fish, milk products, and other types of foods, but the question that arises is: are all of these foods good for us when they are eaten all the time? Which foods are most nutritious and offer the most benefit to our health and quality of life?

A quick reminder about the abuse of unhealthy foods and the consequences that arise from this is the state of health in the developed world. Foods that we can now eat - like fast foods, refined foods, calorically very dense foods (foods that will definitely help us avoid hunger and starvation) - can become deadly if we rely too much on them. Commercial food industries have created a huge amount of food to choose from on a scale that has never been seen before. The greater the choice, the higher the chance of a sale, but that huge choice has also created the emergence of a very harmful trait: foods with long shelf life.

As we all know, food in its natural raw state cannot last very long. Vegetables and fruit, as well as meats and fish, can only last for a few days before they start fermenting or putrefying. Unfortunately, these types of foods are not the staple foods in our diet any more. They have been replaced with various substitutes that have longer shelf lives, that are easier to preserve, to transport, and to store and are therefore more profitable for the companies that create them. Foods that had previously been the only choice on the "menu" for millions of years have now become just a side dish in most cases.

More and more, natural, non-commercially designed food can't be found in the daily menu of the majority of people in developed countries. Products such as pasta, rice, bread, sugar, different types and shapes of grains, and dried, cooked, frozen and tinned edibles have become the main choices of today's modern families. Food which is cheap, easy to buy, easy to prepare, easy to chew, etc. has become the favoured food. But in order to be cheap, and have a long preservation and shelf life, this food has to be totally denatured and pumped with many different chemicals and flavourings in order to resemble something akin to its original shape and taste. Just look for example at a typical box of morning cereal, which is the most common breakfast choice for millions of people. Apart from some processed grains that have lost all links with the living plant they came from, you will see that the content of that box is sugar, cocoa powder, extra vitamins and minerals, flavourings, colours, salt, preservatives and other chemicals. The simple question is: "Why is all this extra stuff needed?" The answer is that most of the natural vitamins, minerals and enzymes have been deactivated (through processing) and lost in exchange for long shelf life. Food should not be reinforced with enzymes, vitamins, minerals and other components that are naturally found in it in the first place. Food should be full of all these components and eaten in a state where all of the nutrients are still present naturally.

So, what would constitute our best dietary choices nowadays? What kind of food would benefit us the most? What do we need to eat in order to stay healthy and energetic, to maintain strength and keep in shape without getting fat? The answers that we are getting from experts usually contradict one another; the perfect foods are either meats, or grains, or some complicated combination of very specific foods, or mathematical calculations or food energy units known as calories. I get bombarded on a daily basis with very scientific and extremely mathematical questions from people who are actually over-weight and very often obese! These people may believe they possess a lot of knowledge, but this knowledge doesn't translate into good health in their own lives. In addition, the average consumer faces a really big problem every time they enter the supermarket - which nutritional guru should they trust and what food should they buy?

This was and still is the most common ground for disagreement among nutritionists, anthropologists and medical professionals. Quite often their professional opinions are biased depending on which of the big food manufacturers they get their financing from. Food manufacturers that spend billions of pounds or dollars on marketing are well aware of the importance of recruiting "qualified" nutritional authorities to expound on the virtues of their products. People need to be convinced that their choice of food is right, they need to hear the evidence that these choices will offer them long life and superior health. This is where the power of "science" can unleash its weapons through the modern mercenaries known as nutritionists, health advisors, dietary consultants, etc.

To make the whole problem of finding the most appropriate foods even more complicated, we have to acknowledge that food has different characteristics which heavily influence the understanding and usage of it among humans. Over time, food has evolved from being just a biological necessity to becoming part of our cultural identifica-tion, a powerful social signal, an economic indicator and an emo-tional commodity. It is very important to understand these different characteristics which influence our eating, in order to understand the causes of overeating, undereating, binge eating, sugar cravings, and preferences for high calorie foods, etc. The phenomenon of eat-ing (either out of necessity or pleasure) is driven by many different forces that can make us very happy and healthy, just as easily as it can do the opposite and make us very unhappy and unhealthy.

The Biological Nature of Food

Many people often wake up in the morning feeling hungry. That feeling of hunger keeps getting stronger and stronger until we satisfy the urge for food by eating. Once we have our breakfast, we feel better, happier, satisfied and ready to roll. This sense of feeling good continues until the point where we get hungry again. We eat again, we feel good again and the pattern repeats itself at least a few times a day. The bottom line is: we eat when we get hungry. However, we should also ask if that is really true for everybody? The answer would be: not really, just for some of us. The feeling of hunger is something that a majority of people regard as a bad feeling, even something unnatural. But looking back on our history we can see that hunger is actually a natural state for humans. We need to be a bit hungry before we eat. Hunger signals that it is time to refuel, that empty space has been created for new food to enter the digestive system. Once the food passes from the first stage of digestion to the next, then we should eat again, but not before that. Digestion is a complicated chemical process that takes place every time food enters our mouth, stomach and small and large intestines. Every meal causes many digestive juices to be released in order to digest macro-nutrients. When the right macronutrients are consumed they create a specific digestive environment that doesn't like to be disrupted with a new influx of food (a new meal) before the first stage of diges-tion (in the stomach) is finished. Putting new food into the stomach before the previous meal has been digested and passed to the small intestine will cause unwanted chemical reactions that will result in bloating, gas, weakened digestion, etc.

Once hunger hits we instinctively eat. That is really great, natural timing! When the body is ready to accept new food, the light feeling of hunger will remind us to eat again. So, one may ask, what is the proper timing between meals? How long do we need to wait before we should eat again? The time gap between meals is determined by many factors such as the amount and type of food eaten in a meal (fat, fibre, water, carbohydrate content), metabolic efficiency, diges-tive efficiency, food cravings etc. It would be very difficult to find perfect rules and expect magically perfect answers like 2 hours, 3 hours or 4 hours. The complexity of digestion and absorption of food doesn't allow for a universal answer that holds for everyone. The only real guidance to perfect timing between meals is the feeling of hunger. Do you get hungry after 2 or 5 hours? The time which has elapsed is completely irrelevant. Hunger has to be the signal that it is time for the next meal. Of course, you should not wait until you are starving; I am referring to that slight onset of hunger that moti-vates you to seek food.

Food is here to give us energy and life. We do eat to live and we should eat when we feel hungry, not before that. Unfortunately, too many of us live to eat and that usually causes us to eat before hunger strikes. First and foremost, we need food to support life. We need food for energy, for the repair of cells and tissues, for strong immunity, for a healthy mental state; these are the main reasons why we have to eat. Without satisfying these basic and natural needs we cannot think about the other characteristics of food. But once we exceed the right amount and type of food needed to satisfy our very basic physiological needs we run into problems.

The Cultural Nature of Food

Being a physiological necessity doesn't mean that food has no other important characteristics. Different foods also reflect our belonging to different groups and cultures. People all around the world have been eating different diets for centuries, identifying their own culture through particular foods and food combinations. People become very proud of their national dishes which have contributed to the development and identity of their national culture. In our modern times, in the developed multicultural world, foods from around the globe have found a place in our everyday menu. We are surrounded by a huge choice of foods from different parts of the world, and diets that have evolved in different cultures and climates. Foods that come from different corners of the globe bring with them large amounts of history, tradition, characteristics and energy which reflect each particular culture. What these foods all have in common is that they are favoured within their specific cultures, and are often seen as the best possible foods to eat. I have come across so many passionate defenders of particular diets from Asia, Africa, America, or from particular countries within these continents. Even the diets from European countries differ drastically, favouring different types and combinations of food that often become proud hallmarks of a given culture or national identity.

Over the centuries, different countries produced different types of foods, mainly influenced by the local climate and geographic variables. Some countries produced more grains, some fruits and vegetables, and some could only grow livestock. But the interesting thing is, wherever people come from, they often maintain the strong belief that their traditional diets are simply the best diets! The typical situation that you see in, for example, multicultural cities is that diets that completely differ from one another are each believed by their defenders to the best ones available.

The cultural nature of food definitely helps people to identify their origins, to gather together, to invoke memories, get closer to each other, strengthen communities, and also to introduce others to their own traditional diets. Introducing others to different traditional foods is one of the many benefits of living in multicultural communities. The diversity of different cultures, without a doubt, makes life more interesting. However, all these positive cultural influences that food is subject to are not guaranties that the traditional diets of different cultures are the healthiest ones.

Worldwide research has proven many times that people in some parts of the world benefit from better health while populations from other corners of the globe suffer much more from chronic diseases. The major difference in their lifestyle is the dietary difference, since they consume different foods and different combinations of foods. Generally speaking, cultures whose diet is composed mainly of vegetables, fruits, fish and lean meats benefit from better health than cultures in which the staple diet is processed foods, high amounts of carbohydrates and lots of saturated and hydrogenated fats.

The Social Nature of Food

Food also plays a big role in different social events, whether a family dinner, wedding, lunch with a group of friends, a night out with a partner, etc. Special occasions and celebrations are all marked by the presentation of food. It is almost impossible to imagine an important social event without the presence of food. Eating together, celebrating together, relaxing and enjoying a special occasion with the accompaniment of food reflects the social importance that food has to human beings.

Although it is a very important characteristic of food that people can benefit from more than the mere biological consequences of eating, the social aspect of food often also drives people to overeat and eat the wrong kinds of food. The problem that is often overlooked in social situations is that any type of food can be overeaten! Whether it is meat, bread, rice, fruit or any combination of these, once overeaten, food creates discomfort, forcing the pancreas to produce large amounts of insulin and causing the food to be stored as body fat. Since we can only digest and absorb a certain amount of food at a time (in a single meal), anything more than that will create digestive difficulties and most likely will end up as unwanted body fat.

Another high calorie "favourite" consumed during social events is alcohol. Alcoholic drinks are the easiest way to ingest huge amounts of calories in a very short time. Easily absorbed, alcohol will almost certainly end up in the body as fat deposits, leading to obesity and being overweight and their attendant and countless health consequences. The "feel good" factor enjoyed during happy and relaxed socialising is not the best way to regulate the right amount and choice of food. This is why it is very important to be aware of the social nature of food and take that into consideration in order to maintain good health while still enjoying social events and occasions.

The Financial Nature of Food

Throughout history we have had situations where poorer classes of people have struggled to survive on very little or low quality food that contained low levels of protein, minerals and/or vitamins. More well-to-do people in society didn't have these problems since gaining access to meat, vegetables and fruits was not usually as difficult for the wealthier members of society. Many illnesses that were widespread among the poor were directly related to the quality and amount of food available to them. Even today, among the poor, we are witnessing higher levels of health problems such as cardiovascular disease, diabetes and obesity, among others.

Good food was almost always available to the wealthy. They, for example, have never suffered from malnutrition and diseases caused by protein deficiency. Some of them may have been overweight (due to over-eating: indulging in sugary and starchy foods), but they have had access to quality food. Financial power was and still is one of the most important factors when it comes to having access to high quality food.

Quality food is not cheap; high quality fruit and vegetables are grown differently, picked at a different stage of ripening and stored differently. Quality meats are reared and matured differently; and overall, producing higher quality food takes longer and costs more money. This is why our quality foods are more expensive. Good quality food (fruits and vegetables) have a higher amount of vitamins and minerals, and the meat of grass-fed animals has a lower level of saturated fat and higher levels of omega-3 oils. Being more "powerful", good quality foods offer better protection against diseases, better health and therefore a better quality of life. In light of all this, the question that arises is: can everyone afford to eat the highest quality food?

Over-population of the species has forced food manufacturers to produce cheaper foods, to produce them faster and to extend their shelf life. This is the only way to manufacture food that can be affordable for the majority of the population. But since cheap food is poorer in quality (while not always poorer in calories), it usually needs to be eaten in larger amounts, causing weight problems and obesity.

Although financial power will never be distributed proportionately amongst everyone in a society, it is still possible to optimise the chances for good health for the majority of people. The way to do this is to avoid eating unnatural foods that have been heavily processed. Those foods are usually full of sugars, processed grains, saturated and hydrogenated fats, salt, additives and other substances that are designed mainly to prolong shelf life.

The Emotional Nature of Food

We all know that our emotional state can heavily influence both our choice of food and the amount of food that we eat. We don't eat the same amount or quality of food in normal everyday circumstances as we do in situations of stress, sadness, loneliness or other emotional disturbances. We tend to eat more when we are bored, lonely, anxious or need to comfort ourselves. Food is a very powerful comfort tool, especially food full of carbohydrates. I have never heard of someone having overeaten steak or fish whilst being in an emotion-ally stressful situation!

Deep inside of us, we all have written memories that date from long ago, collective memories that, over time, turn into instincts. For most of our evolution, food was relatively scarce and any important events (which didn't happen very often) would be celebrated by eat-ing more than usual. Our instinct for survival drove us towards con-suming calorie-dense foods. The higher the caloric intake, the more energy would be ingested and the higher the chances for survival would be. This is the reason why we have developed the taste for fat and sugary food, the foods that in harsh living conditions would offer us the highest chance of survival. So it is understandable why, during a time of emotional distress, we choose food that is rather high in calories. In order to comfort ourselves, we unconsciously try to protect ourselves.

Emotional disturbances often make us vulnerable and endangered. Usually the only power we have in moments of fear and loneliness is the power to eat. It is during these times that we exploit our only dominance. We eat to protect ourselves, to please ourselves and to feel good. While we eat we do feel good and are pleased and comforted.

The best way to control unpredictable and unwanted eating binges then is to reconsider our own lifestyle. In order to lower the possibil-ity of difficult emotional situations we have to engage in identify-ing our goals (short-term, medium-term and long-term) in all areas of life and strive to achieve them. If we are satisfied and fulfilled through the achievement of our goals, we are more likely to improve our chances of avoiding emotional difficulties.

The bottom line

- Natural food doesn't last long on the shelf due to the high content of life boosting enzymes. In order to preserve food and extend its shelf life, manufacturers have to denature the food and create edibles that are highly processed and free of enzymes.
- In order to live healthily, eat to live, do not live to eat.
- Do not eat before you feel hungry; hunger is a natural signal that the body is ready to eat.
- Not all traditional diets are necessarily healthy.
- It's very easy to overeat during social events.
- Everyone can benefit from eating less processed food full of sugars and starches, and eating more natural foods.
- Emotional disturbances are known to cause overeating particularly of unhealthy types of food.

The Legacy of Evolution

Food that has been available to us throughout most of our evolution is no longer part of our staple diet. Whilst a large variety of animal and plant foods have been on our menu for hundreds of thousands of years, food that comprises the bulk of what is consumed nowadays in the western world is based mainly on a few different types of grains. Although grains are not part of the original natural food that we have evolved around (they were introduced into our diet relatively recently with the discovery of agriculture), we still denature grain foods before consumption. Before they are ready to be eaten nowadays, we strip them of all the goodness that unprocessed grains might still bring. Refined grains constitute our staple food in the form of bread, cereals, rice, pasta, cakes, sweets and similar products. Composed of pure (tasteless) starch, refined grains are often pumped with different types of simple sugars in order to improve their taste, giving them even higher caloric density. We are consuming foods that never existed before, and the amount of calories that we are eating daily due to these unnatural edibles is many times higher than we have ever eaten in the past.

For most of our evolution we have been hunters and gatherers, consuming primarily meat, roots, vegetables, fruits, seeds and nuts, all in their natural state. The natural state of these foods means that they still possess all the important micronutrients, enzymes and fibres in the perfect amount and balance for optimal digestion and health at the time that they are eaten. Most of the food that people eat today is denatured, devoid of the original micronutrients that are essential for health. During previous periods in our evolution, our anatomy and physiology had been accustomed to and perfectly adapted to this type of food. For some millions of years, our predecessors have managed to survive on plant foods and meat by successfully adapting their physiology and anatomy to them. Bearing in mind that the last ice age spread through a period beginning some 70 000 years ago and finishing some 10 000 years ago, it wouldn't be wrong to conclude that during that time, humans managed to survive mainly on available meats and seafood instead of plants! Not many plants would grow in those climatic extremes. Neither grains nor products made from them existed during our adaptation to what was predominant in our natural environment for so much of our development. And before grains were introduced into the human diet, humans had evolved perfectly. According to the latest archaeological studies, we are still the same humans (physiologically and anatomically) that existed 190 000 years ago!

The major difference between our ancestors and us (in terms of nutrition) is in the selection and types of food that we eat. For most of our history, finding food required a big effort, so our ancestors mainly ate to live. All they were doing was hunting and gathering in order to survive. Eating one day would mean having a few more days of livelihood afterwards. Life simply depended on eating.

Today, most of us live to eat! We rarely eat only when we are hungry, and most of us never experience "real" hunger any more. A little hunger naturally activates a major panic button; everything has to stop and we have to eliminate the most unexpected and surprising feeling that people in developed countries can experience nowadays. However, today we use any little excuse to justify our eating. We don't eat only because we are hungry, we eat because it is time to eat, because there is a social event, because we are bored, because we are happy or we are depressed, because others are eating, etc… We simply see eating as the most powerful tool to comfort ourselves. And when food becomes a medication for improving our emotional state or a way of expressing our social belonging, we lose respect towards food; we forget that food is what gives us life and as such should be understood and approached on a different level.

If we respected food more, we would choose better food and we would eat enough but no more; we wouldn't overeat. If we respected food we would respect ourselves more and we wouldn't eat everything that we can put in our mouths. We would eat food that has been given to us by nature, a non-profitable establishment; not products that have been created in order to raise profits, backed by people who like to be called scientists and who have never learned the basics of the history of life, evolution, anthropology or physiology. We wouldn't trust people who would sell anything in order to make a profit, like celebrities that advertise shaving creams one day and then food the next, or journalists who report on wars one day and then about "healthy" diets the next.

Fake food needs marketing and advertising, it needs to be explained and introduced to the general public. The main reason for this is that thousands of new food products are introduced to the market every year, products that never existed before and are totally unknown to us. They are usually reinforced with some "super" micronutrients like vitamin C, iron, B12, omega-3 fatty acids or something else in order to gain more credibility and market value. Billions are spent every year on food marketing! Just ask yourself: when did you last see an advert for fresh vegetables, fruit, meat or fish?

Natural food just needs to be eaten, as it has been for millions of years. We have situations today where people don't eat fruits and vegetables for weeks or even months at a time! Wondering what they do eat? Edibles made by food industries, edibles resembling natural, real food which are coloured and flavoured to do so. They eat products that have to be pumped with vitamins and minerals, because these products are devoid of them, pumped with enzymes because they have been lost through cooking, freezing and drying. Most people eat edibles that have to be made or dressed up, rather than nature's ready-made foods. These are edibles that I call dead foods.

In order to boost sales, manufacturers of processed foods have been trying for some time to enrich the same empty food with vitamins, minerals, fibre and proteins, making them seem more attractive and "natural". Extra fibre into yoghurt, white bread (making it "whole-meal") and cereals; extra vitamins and minerals into butter, bread, milk, cereals and other foods; extra protein into sausages and other cheap meat products (as well as products for vegetarians), etc. The food industry is merely acting out of desperation to improve some-thing that cannot be improved. Junk food, fortified with synthetic vitamins and minerals and cheap protein substitutes, will still be empty junk food. To make matters worse, very often the wrong ingredients end up in the wrong place: omega-3 fatty acids in milk and eggs, vitamins D and A in cereals, calcium in fruit juices, fibre in yoghurt, and many other ingredients artificially placed where they simply don't belong. These micronutrients naturally occur in totally different foods! Omega-3 is found in oily ocean fish, not in eggs; calcium is found in dark green vegetables, not in orange juice; and fibre is found in fruit and vegetables, not in milk! Regardless, food manufacturers will try to impress you with these Frankenstein com-binations in order to gain access to your pockets.

We are witnessing more and more of these immoral attempts to create perfect edibles that try to resemble natural foods. Natural foods are so perfect in their composition and effect on the human body that it is simply impossible to create something from heavily processed ingredients that will even come close to the natural concept. Fortifying processed food with different micro and macro elements is the best proof of how many essential components have been removed during the numerous stages of processing.

Natural foods are high in water content, high in fibre, high in vitamins and minerals. Processed foods are low in water content, low in fibre and low in vitamins and minerals. These huge differences between food that nature has miraculously created for us and greed-driven, processed food products are the major reason for our poor responses to those processed foods, and have resulted in chronic diseases that were unknown until 10 000 years ago.

Our ancestors enjoyed a life free of chronic diseases, as do all indigenous cultures around the world that have preserved traditional ways of living and eating. Their diets have been much richer in essential minerals, vitamins, omega-3 fatty acids, protein, enzymes, fibre and water, while being low in refined carbohydrates.

The bottom line

- Our staple foods today are made mainly from refined grains that have been stripped of all of the goodness that unrefined grains provide.

- Thanks to heavy processing of grains, our daily caloric intake is many times over that of our ancestors, who were hunters and gatherers and didn't eat grains.
- The staple foods that allowed our ancestors freedom from chronic diseases were composed of meat, fruits and vegetables, seeds and nuts.
- Natural food is full of fibre, vitamins, minerals and enzymes. Processed, denatured food is often "enriched" with extra vitamins and minerals in order to emulate the power of natural foods.
- Trying to recreate natural food from dead, denatured ingredients is never good for our health.

Food - Health

For most people today, health has never been understood to its fullest depth and meaning. Because of this, most of us realize the importance of it only in times of sickness and poor health. When something starts hurting, we remember how nice it was when we didn't experience any pain or discomfort, how nice it was when we were healthy. However, the absence of illness in itself shouldn't be confused with being healthy! Health is more than that; health is the overall optimised mental and physical state in which an individual can explore all the options of human creativity: intellectual, social, artistic, spiritual etc. We, the people of the 21st century, know very well that without a balanced life in its most basic form, our health will be at risk.

Unhappiness and a lack of fulfilment are most often the first causes of unhealthy mental conditions. Depression is one of these mental conditions with which a lot of people are familiar. The complexity of our mental and physical ethos provides a lot of room for the existence of psychosomatic conditions, which are conditions in which mental disturbances can cause physical conditions and vice versa. All of this should suggest that the proper balance between all our life forces is the condition we know as "health".

The proper balance of our life forces is something that is not just inherited (the balance between our mental and physical well-being), it is something that develops from an early age and has to continue to develop throughout our lifetime. In most cases, in a way, good health is a product of our own personal balance! We can continue to support that good health, a necessary condition for life, that the majority of us receive from birth. Health awareness is the most powerful reason to engage in a lifestyle that will allow us to optimise all our human potentials and continue to maintain good health throughout our lifetime.

A lifestyle that, among other important factors, incorporates positive attitudes, healthy eating and regular exercise will offer much greater opportunity for good health. In this holistic approach, the food that we consume is one of the most important factors that will maintain and support our health.

If we look at the physical aspects of human health we again discover that the synergy (perfect balance) of our body systems is a pre-requisite of good health. Each bodily system has to deliver a certain level of efficiency in precise balance with all the others. The cardio-vascular system, for example, has to perform with certain efficiency in order to allow the transport of oxygen to every cell in the body. Only with an efficient respiratory system is this possible. If the lungs don't function efficiently enough to supply the blood with adequate amounts of oxygen, we will experience many problems in the form of poor health. If, for example, the hormonal system fails to deliver, a disruption of many different metabolic processes in the body will occur, followed by problems of the cardiac system (along with other undesirable consequences). Inefficient elimination of the by-products of digestion will cause the build up of toxins in the body and overstress the immune system. All of these things make it very clear that the food we eat is the single most powerful thing that influences our health.

Food shouldn't be thought of only as the sum of necessary calories and essential nutrients, but also as a very powerful medicine! Food has the important ability to trigger different hormonal responses that will further cause other important biochemical responses in the body. However, those hormonal reactions can be either positive or negative. It's entirely our decision which type of hormonal responses we will create by consuming different foods. Bearing in mind that a hormonal reaction is the precursor of all other bodily reactions and functions, we should never forget the power of food to orchestrate the balance of all our bodily systems.

Eating bread was never and will never be the same as eating meat. Bread causes a totally different hormonal response in the body and its digestion requires the production of different enzymes than the digestion of meat. Eating meat will create different hormonal reactions and will cause a completely different digestive environment than eating bread. Whilst bread is still a new and unknown food to our physiology, meat is the food that humans have been eating for hundred of thousands of years and have evolved around.

Over-consumption of carbohydrates will force the body to produce more of a particular hormone, insulin, and less of other hormones, for example glucagon. This also puts more stress on the pancreas, the internal gland that produces insulin. Storing more body fat – which is a direct consequence of the over-consumption of carbohydrates and the related over-production of insulin – puts more stress on the skeletal system because of the extra body weight. By increasing body weight with extra body fat you will also put additional stress on the cardiovascular and other systems. Eating the wrong foods, or merely overeating, can easily create a whole set of unwanted chain reactions.

By controlling the amount and type of food that we eat on a daily basis, we can create a positive hormonal response and therefore a positive balance for all our body systems. A positive balance of all body systems is the right environment for good health and proper food is the most important criterion for meeting this goal.

Eating habits have been heavily overlooked in modern lifestyle theories. Eating has been seen rather as a cultural or social phenomenon, while the natural aspect of it has been completely forgotten. That has created a culture of overeaters, binge eaters and blind followers of "celebrity chefs". Living in the world of taste extravaganza we have forgotten to give the advantage to good food, and instead we have become slaves of different spices and seasonings! Being bombarded with sugar, salt and other extremely powerful spices, most of us have already lost the taste for healthy food. When it comes to the degree of sweetness, apples and pears will definitely lose the battle against sweets and cakes.

Eating for pleasure or out of boredom, when taste becomes the only sense guiding us through the process, is the best possible scenario for becoming overweight, obese, diabetic and also prone to many cardiovascular diseases, as well as some types of cancer.

Our health directly depends on our way of eating: our selection of food and the amount of food that we eat. Non-biological reasons for eating, which have never before been discussed seriously, have become the main obstacle to our health. We in the developed world have completely displaced the role of food in our lives. Instead of respecting nature's original intention that we should eat in order to live, we have effectively started living in order to eat nowadays! Food has become the main goal, not the life that we live.

The consequences of this misplaced goal are very expensive and we pay the price in the form of reduced health and happiness. Food must not become the first or only satisfaction that people strive for in their lives. When the power to eat anything at any time becomes the dominant one in someone's life, it creates a complex psychological problem. Achieving happiness and fulfilment cannot happen only through putting food in our mouth! In a balanced lifestyle, where other human needs are fulfilled in the correct order, eating fulfils a life-supporting role rather than a life-ruling role. In the balanced lifestyle scenario, obsession with food does not occur and good health can be preserved for longer periods, enabling us to enjoy all the happiness that life can bring.

The complexity of modern living has created a lifestyle that has re-sulted in poor health for a high percentage of the population. Eating habits have changed and contributed towards the development of an eating culture that we recognize today through binge eating, eating non-nutritious fast foods, and the heavy absence of fruits, vegetables and quality protein in our diets. We strive for calorically-dense foods, for foods that we don't need to chew, and foods that we don't have to spend time preparing. Our eating experience today revolves mainly around detecting the taste of sugar, salt and exotic spices. Absolutely everything, from baby food to everyday food and food for special occasions, has to be heavily sugared, salted and spiced in order to satisfy our taste buds!

We have lost the ability to recognize food that does us good and sup-ports our health through proper hormonal balance, an efficient cardio-vascular system, strong skeletal system, etc. The only way to return to natural communication with food and reoptimise our life is to become informed and motivated, and then make a difference by taking action.

Unfortunately, our knowledge about food didn't come from an understanding of what good food can do for us, but instead through what bad food has done to us. After finally understanding that the single biggest cause of all chronic diseases (currently the number one cause of death) is the poor food that has become our staple diet, we have finally learned what we should eat in order to protect and strengthen our health. Although we have learned it the hard way, there are still many obstacles to having this knowledge accepted by the general public.

The bottom line

- Food is not the simple sum of calories and nutrients, food is also a very powerful medicine.
- Food triggers the response of many important hormones in the body.
- The synergy of our bodily systems is influenced by the food that we eat.
- A taste for fresh and natural food is essential for our long term health.

Chronic Diseases

In this chapter I will help you to understand the link between food
and chronic diseases. For some reason, the medical establishment is
still very reluctant to spell out the major cause of the largest killers
of modern times, chronic diseases. Most chronic diseases are self-
inflicted and are directly related to the food that we eat. Constantly
bombarding all the body's systems with the wrong kind of food from
birth onwards seldom results in a happy ending. It is entirely up to
our genetic predisposition just how long someone who has been eating improperly from an early age will manage to live in good health.
Luckier ones will live disease-free for longer, the less lucky ones
will start suffering earlier. One way or another, most of us will end
up with some form of chronic disease before we reach the age of 50.
Interestingly though, chronic diseases were not part of the human experience for most of our evolution. Chronic diseases first appeared
in human history along with the introduction of grains in our diets,
some 10 000 years ago. For millions of years before that, during
the period that we evolved around the food responsible for creating
our physiology, our bodies were always capable of preserving good
health. The food that was available before the introduction of grains
never led to any chronic diseases.

Just like any other mammal (mammals living in natural environments
that is, not ones reared by humans), we have consistently eaten only
particular types of foods for hundreds of thousands of years. As a
result of this, we were blessed with great health prior to the discovery
of agriculture. Remains of humans dating from before this time (older
than 10 000 years) are the best proof that diseases such as tooth decay,

cardiovascular diseases, diabetes, bone deformities and other diseases of modern times didn't exist then. Even in the modern day, cultures that still live as hunters and gatherers in remote parts of the world have no chronic diseases!

Enjoying the benefits of civilisation doesn't have to mean that a heavy price has to be attached to eating. The benefits of modern technologies can be enjoyed without necessarily being unhealthy for us. The basic practices of our modern lifestyle have to be reconsidered and the priorities changed in order to continue to develop without losing one of the most essential fundamentals: health. It is entirely our choice, as much an individual choice as a collective one.

The causes of chronic disease have been very well known to both the scientific community and the general public for a long time now. Although the information has been available to every one of us in one form or another, not much has changed over time. The fact is that chronic diseases are constantly increasing globally. Millions of people are dying around the world due to chronic diseases caused primarily by a poor lifestyle. Improper diets composed mostly of food that we have never gotten used to, and a lack of physical activity are the major causes of diabetes, cardiovascular problems, cancer, allergies, tooth decay, bone deformities and many other medical conditions that are killing us globally by the many millions every year. The medical establishments around the world are not explicit enough in pointing to the major causes of chronic diseases. Improper foods are still the staple of the majority of people's diets, and although statistics are pointing to higher life expectancy in developed countries, we never hear about the quality of life, which is the optimised functioning of all body systems in perfect synergy - definitely not on the agenda of modern politicians, scientists or medical experts.

A good quality of life would require, among other things, an absence of chronic disease which would only be possible if the right diet and adequate physical activity regained their correct place in human life. Our anatomy and physiology should be our only guide in the search for a perfect human diet and perfect physical engagement.

The constant race for profit has put big industries which directly influence our lifestyle (food, health supplements, fashion, fitness, etc.) in constant competition against each other. A completely distorted picture has thus emerged from this. Fashion, trends, habits, social acceptance and other powerful factors heavily influence the everyday life of millions of people. Life in its essence, being the synergy of optimised life functions, has become a tool rather than a goal because of the constant war for profit. Instead of using the benefits of different technologies and advances of modern civilisation in general to optimise our human experience (higher quality of life through enhanced intellectual, moral and physical existence), we are blindly following the logic of profit, which has quite a damaging effect on our health.

Everything would be fine if we could easily cope with the denaturalisation of human life, which includes such things as fast foods, binge eating, drinking, smoking, taking drugs, inactivity, etc. But we don't. Only superficially have we adapted to the pace and trends of modern life; statistics keep screaming at us that we have never really adapted to this situation. Anatomically, physiologically and mentally, we will most likely never adapt to the modern lifestyle that has overtaken our time-tested natural lifestyle which was slowly developed over millions of years.

Although modern medicine seems to be able to solve the majority of the health consequences caused by our inadequate lifestyles (or more

precisely it calms them down), we are still silently accepting defeat.
It seems that we are powerless to defend our own human ethos
against the dark side of our nature, represented by greed and laziness
Chronic diseases are still the biggest killers of human beings right
now. They are all the consequence of an incorrect lifestyle, domi-
nated by unhealthy eating and inactivity, with a large majority of
individual cases of illness being self-inflicted.

The most widespread conditions that are ruining human health these
days are hypertension, high cholesterol levels in the blood, insulin
resistance and diabetes, or different combinations of these. In order
to understand the link between their causes and human nutrition, we
need to look at all of the conditions we have just mentioned.

Hypertension (High Blood Pressure)

High blood pressure is the primary cause of cardiovascular problems
including fatal heart attacks. High blood pressure has been treated
as a disease and is usually treated with medication. It can often be
reduced, but not eliminated, because the major causes of high blood
pressure are never considered, properly assessed and treated. Instead
of finding the causes and eliminating them in order to stop the consequences, high blood pressure (a symptom in itself) is treated and
lowered on a daily basis, which is concrete confirmation that only
the symptom is being treated and not the cause. If the causes of the
problem were tackled and eradicated, daily treatments for the rest of
the patient's life would not be necessary. Untreated causes require
treatment of the consequences for life and, unfortunately, this is the
current situation in modern medical philosophy: treating the symptoms but not the cause! This is why hypertension has been regarded

as a disease, while in fact it is a symptom of a different problem, not the cause itself, and therefore not a disease in its own right.

In order to understand this condition it is necessary to understand the underlying causes of high blood pressure and the possibility of eliminating the same. Only by eliminating the causes of hypertension is it possible to eliminate the condition itself. As the title of this book suggests, the domain of nutrition will be examined in order to discover any connections between the food that we eat, our response to it, and the causes of hypertension. The best possible scenario would be the ability to correct the causes of high blood pressure with a simple change in our diet. Let us see how this is possible.

There are several major causes of high blood pressure, but in this book we will focus on two causes in particular which are of direct interest to us: fluid retention and thickening of the arteries. Both of these causes are mainly due to the same risk factor and represent the consequences of the most neglected and underestimated disease: hyper-production of insulin.

Fluid Retention/Hyperproduction of Insulin

Insulin is a hormone produced by the pancreas. Its main role is to transport glucose (blood sugar) from the blood to cells throughout the body. It is one of the most essential hormones and is produced every time we eat. In our digestive system, food gets broken down into different particles (protein, fat, carbohydrates), carbohydrates being the major trigger of insulin production. Therefore, the more carbohydrates we eat (in the form of bread, rice, pasta, sweets, cakes, etc.) the more insulin we produce. Eating more carbohydrates creates more glucose in the blood, which in turn requires more insulin to lower it and transport it to where energy is stored in the body. There are two major stores of energy in the body: glycogen stored in the liver and muscle tissues, and fat, which is stored in various locations. In the case of saturated glycogen stores, our bodies convert any extra blood sugar into body fat. Everything functions properly when there is adequate caloric intake, selection of foods, and adequate and efficient daily activity.

A problem arises, however, when the previously mentioned circumstances are not met. When we eat more than we should, when we eat the wrong food, and when we are not active enough, we find ourselves in complete biochemical havoc! Eating too much of the wrong food will produce too much blood sugar, forcing the production of a huge amount of insulin in order to lower the blood sugar level to a safe and acceptable one. Inactivity will keep the glycogen stores full, because they cannot be emptied without vigorous daily physical activity (resistance training being the most effective). When the glycogen stores in the muscles and liver are full, extra blood sugar is driven by insulin into the body's fat stores. This is a very simple way to get fat! The hyperproduction of insulin can be very damaging, especially if it occurs daily. Due to modern lifestyles and the lack of knowledge about healthy eating and fitness, daily overproduction of insulin is extremely common, resulting in one-way traffic of extra glucose from the blood into the body's fat deposits.

Insulin production is related to the issue of hypertension; insulin is the hormone that forces the kidneys to retain more sodium. More sodium in the body causes more fluid retention, which directly increases the amount of blood and therefore causes an increase in blood pressure. When insulin is over-produced, due to an inactive lifestyle and an inappropriate diet (a diet high in carbohydrates and low in protein and fibre), the amount of sodium continues to rise causing the retention of more and more fluid and therefore higher blood pressure. Over time, untreated high blood pressure can cause serious heart problems, including heart attacks.

Thickening of the Arteries/Hyperproduction of Insulin

When the arterial walls thicken and become more rigid and less flexible, blood flow slows down. In order to deliver the right amount of blood to every part of the body in a timely fashion, the heart has to pump harder, which increases the pressure on the arterial walls and results in elevated blood pressure. There are many factors that cause the thickening of the arteries, but the most relevant to the subject of this book are the effects of insulin and high cholesterol.

Insulin is a hormone with strong anabolic properties. Not only skeletal muscles grow under the influence of insulin, but smooth muscle tissues too. Arteries, being made of smooth muscle tissues, thicken under the influence of the hyper-production of insulin. Too much consumption of carbohydrates causes exactly that; over-production of insulin which affects the blood flow through the narrowed arteries caused by thickening of arterial smooth muscle tissue. Correcting daily eating habits is the most successful way to manage the over-production of insulin in the body.

Another factor that causes narrowing of the arteries is the build-up of cholesterol on the arterial walls. This cholesterol, in combination with other fats, proteins and minerals, creates plaque deposits that can become permanent, causing terminal narrowing of the arteries. Narrowing of the arteries causes a rise in blood pressure, which affects the heart and kidneys accordingly. An excess of insulin also increases cholesterol production, which results in increased blood pressure. Again, the combination of the right diet and an effective exercise program is the best long-term solution in the prevention of and fight against the consequences of excessive cholesterol production.

Preventing and curing high blood pressure is possible and achievable through healthy eating and adequate physical exercise. However, the administration of different types of medications in order to eliminate or lower blood pressure, without any changes in diet and activities, is unfortunately the current line of attack for the majority of sufferers of high blood pressure. Without a change in lifestyle any treatment, including medical treatments, can only temporarily mask the problem and will never eliminate its cause. Eliminating the cause of the problem is the ultimate victory over deadly hypertension and is only achievable through altering our dietary and exercise habits. A diet relatively low in carbohydrates and high in protein, essential fats, and fibre, complemented by resistance training, is the best way to prevent high blood pressure and can also cure a majority of cases.

High Cholesterol

High cholesterol levels in the blood contribute to the creation of plaque on the arterial walls, narrowing the passage for the blood to flow through the arteries, thereby increasing blood pressure and causing other cardiovascular problems. Over time this plaque can calcify and become permanent, causing a major risk to the heart.

Before further investigating the danger of high cholesterol presence in the blood, let us first examine the nature and importance of cholesterol in the body. Contrary to popular belief, cholesterol is not fat. It is a waxy, solid alcohol that is produced in every single cell in the body. The fact that every cell can produce cholesterol shows what an essential role cholesterol plays in the life of a cell. Although every cell can produce it, most of them depend on the cholesterol produced in the liver, intestines and skin. Cholesterol directly regulates the viscosity of the cell membrane, regulating the passage of absorbed nutrients into the cell and the pace of removing waste products from the cell into the inter-cellular space. When a cell membrane becomes too soft, allowing more traffic than necessary, the cell produces more cholesterol to adjust the rigidity of the membrane. When the membrane has a higher rigidity than needed, cholesterol is removed from the membrane in order to correct the situation and better facilitate the two-way traffic of nutrients and waste products.

Some of the most important hormones in the body, such as testosterone and oestrogen, are made from cholesterol. These sex hormones are essential to many important life functions, and without enough cholesterol there would not be enough of these essential chemical messengers. Aldosterone, the hormone responsible for sodium regulation in the body and therefore instrumental in the maintenance of healthy blood pressure, is also made out of cholesterol, as is hydrocortisone, the body's natural steroid.

Vitamin D, essential for the absorption of calcium, is produced from cholesterol in the skin. If there is a lack of cholesterol for this purpose, the normal metabolism of calcium will be disturbed, due to the lack of vitamin D in the body. Cholesterol in the skin also regulates the hydration of the skin and protects it from cracking and infections.

These important roles of cholesterol in the body suggest that it is indeed essential for human health. Without sufficient amounts of cholesterol on a daily basis the body's health will deteriorate.

Cholesterol is transported around the body by the blood in the form of lipoproteins. Lipoproteins are a combination of protein and cholesterol. There are several types of lipoprotein, but we will concentrate on the two most important, LDL and HDL. LDL stands for Low Density Lipoprotein, and is commonly referred to as "bad cholesterol". LDL carries more cholesterol than all other types of lipoproteins as it is literally made up entirely of cholesterol. LDL transports cholesterol to the outlaying tissues and, although it can be reabsorbed and used by the liver or other tissues, LDL can also deposit cholesterol on the walls of the arteries.

HDL stands for High Density Lipoprotein, also known as "good cholesterol", and its main role is to take cholesterol from the arterial walls and transfer it back to the liver where it is stored. The actions of LDL and HDL occur simultaneously and the balance between them determines the destiny of cholesterol in the body. More LDL in the blood means that more cholesterol is deposited within the arteries. When there is more HDL in the blood, more cholesterol is transferred in the opposite direction. The right ratio between LDL and HDL is of vital importance to good health.

Since the need for cholesterol is decided within each individual cell in the body, the amount of cholesterol which circulates in the blood directly depends on the regulatory functions within the cellular system. If the cells decide to take more cholesterol from the blood, there will be less free cholesterol in the bloodstream that can be deposited on the walls of the arteries and therefore less risk of heart disease. This would be the perfect scenario. If the cells for some reason produce more than enough cholesterol themselves, less cholesterol will be taken from the bloodstream and more cholesterol will be left floating in the blood, most likely ending up deposited on the interior walls of the arteries. Knowing that, can we do anything to instruct our cells to take more cholesterol from the blood and lower the potential risk of cholesterol deposits within the arteries? Is there anything that can perhaps be done with a proper diet? Well, the answer is YES. Only with the proper diet can we control our hormonal balance, causing our body cells to harvest the cholesterol from the blood and lower the overall amount of LDL in favour of HDL, providing the correct ratio between the two.

Once again, there are two major hormones that will determine the destiny of cholesterol in our body: insulin and glucagon. Whilst insulin stimulates higher production of cholesterol within the cells and therefore less demand for cholesterol from outside them, increasing the overall amount of cholesterol in the blood, glucagon does exactly the opposite. It stimulates the cells to open the receptors responsible for taking cholesterol from outside and from LDL. Under the influence of glucagon, cells use more cholesterol from LDL and produce less themselves, thereby lowering the amount of LDL and lessening the risk of cholesterol deposits on the arterial walls.

To simplify the situation, more insulin will create more LDL and more health risk, while more glucagon will reduce the amount of LDL and lower the risk of cholesterol deposits. The only way to decrease and normalise insulin production is to reduce the overall intake of carbohydrates in the diet. Increased amounts of protein, combined with a reduction of carbohydrates in the diet, ultimately increase the production of glucagon and balance the blood sugar level by stimulating higher absorption of cholesterol from the blood. This is yet another example of how a diet high in protein and fibre, and relatively low in carbohydrates, can reduce the presence of cholesterol and LDL in the blood and maintain or increase the amount of HDL.

Research has shown that diets low in carbohydrates, even when high in fat, can improve the overall cholesterol balance in the body. Since dietary fat doesn't affect insulin production, but rather increases the amount of HDL in the absence of carbohydrates and presence of protein, it has for decades been wrongly blamed for increased cholesterol damage to the body.

Although the factors that can cause elevated cholesterol levels are numerous and include genetics (if your parents have suffered from high cholesterol you should regularly check yours), age (high cholesterol is often associated with older age), gender (men suffer from high cholesterol more often than women), body weight (people who are overweight tend to have higher blood cholesterol), and stress, it appears that elevated insulin always makes the cholesterol problem worse.

A diet low in carbohydrates, particularly simple sugars, and high in protein, fibre and essential fats keeps insulin within the normal range and stimulates production of glucagons. At the same time this same diet will lower the amount of LDL, which is responsible for deadly cholesterol deposits within the arteries, and increase the amount of HDL, which is responsible for the cleaning of cholesterol deposits from the arteries.

Healthy dietary habits are recommended as the preferable way to control insulin and bad cholesterol in the blood, instead of medications that are, in most cases, prescribed only to eliminate the consequences rather than the root causes of these health problems. Only by preventing the causes of health problems or eliminating the existing ones through diet and exercise can good health be achieved and maintained.

Diabetes

Diabetes is a condition that is constantly on the rise. Being a relatively new health condition to the human race, diabetes has a lot to do with poor diet and lifestyle, especially in its milder form, type 2 diabetes.

Although diabetes was discovered some 2 000 years ago, only seventy years ago it was believed that there was only one form of this disease. The major symptoms of diabetic patients are frequent urination, constant thirst, and high levels of sugar in the urine. Whilst they have more or less the same symptoms, different causes distinguish the two different types of diabetes: type 1 and type 2.

Type 1 diabetes develops early in life, in childhood or adolescence, and is more severe than type 2. Its development is caused by the pancreas's inability to produce insulin due to a virus, a toxic substance, or one's immune system destroying the islets of Langerhans, the pancreatic cells that produce insulin. Patients suffering from type 1 diabetes must receive insulin injections in order to metabolise sugar properly. Without the presence of insulin death is certain.

Type 2 diabetes develops in adulthood. Whilst the first symptom of type 1 diabetes is sudden weight loss, type 2 diabetes usually starts with weight gain! This suggests that the development of these two types of diabetes follows different paths. Whilst type 1 diabetes is due to a lack of insulin, type 2 diabetes is caused by excess insulin.

Type 2 diabetes begins with a condition known as insulin resistance. This is when cells refuse to accept glucose driven by insulin because their insulin receptors have become resistant. In this situation, when there is more sugar in the blood, the body produces even more insulin, increasing insulin resistance further. More insulin is produced, but high blood sugar remains, causing the same problems as high blood sugar in type 1 diabetes: high blood pressure, high cholesterol levels, heart disease and, in the later stages, damage to the kidneys, eyes and nerves. In addition, blood circulation in the lower limbs can be affected. Type 2 diabetes is a consequence of insulin inefficiency. In many cases this condition can be successfully treated with simply the right diet and exercise, which increase insulin sensitivity. In some cases, type 2 diabetes has to be controlled by insulin tablets or injections.

When we examine the basic nature of diabetes it becomes apparent that the insulin problem is what has to be solved in both types of diabetes. Whilst the consequences of type 1 diabetes can be eased through better nutrition, insulin resistance (glucose intolerance) can also be successfully controlled by healthy eating, which ultimately means lowering the insulin level by reducing the body's intake of the ultimate insulin provocateur, carbohydrates. A diet low in carbohydrates and high in protein, essential fats, water and fibre is once again the best solution for sufferers of types 1 or 2 diabetes, and at the same time is the best way to prevent insulin resistance. One must note, however, that due to the complex nature of diabetes, diabetics should receive constant medical supervision even in the case of proper food selection and diet.

These three major chronic diseases (perhaps better seen as consequences of different unhealthy causes) - high blood pressure, high
cholesterol level and diabetes - are major causes of serious health
problems that result in hundreds of thousands of deaths annually.
These three diseases in themselves cause two other major diseases;
heart disease and obesity.

This book aims to improve the understanding of healthy eating and
the powerful influence of food on the major hormones of the body,
and therefore discussions and analyses of chronic diseases will be
limited to only a few. Instead, we will concentrate on the major
causes of those diseases as they relate to the main subject of nutrition.
Before going further, a short review of heart disease in relation to the
previously mentioned chronic diseases, and their prevention and cure
through healthy eating, deserves a closer look.

Heart Disease

Heart disease is primarily caused by the disrupted supply of oxygen
and other essential nutrients to the heart muscle. As the body's most
important and hardest working muscle (it works constantly throughout one's life), the heart contains many blood vessels that supply
oxygenated blood to all parts of the body. When a disruption of
blood supply occurs through cholesterol build up on the arterial walls
or thickening of these walls (caused by hyperproduction of insulin),
part of the heart will eventually die and the muscle itself will be in
serious trouble.

In order to keep coronary arteries open and supple, it is necessary to
prevent their clotting and thickening. This can be achieved via two

practices, healthy eating and regular (daily) exercise. These practices will increase blood flow and strengthen the heart muscle at the same time.

Healthy eating involves implementing a diet that will not greatly increase insulin production, because it is rich in protein and essential fats, fibre and water, but low in carbohydrates. Only wholesome, natural food will offer us all the benefits of a healthy heart. The right amount of vitamins and minerals, proteins, fats, carbohydrates, fibre and water available in healthy food is what the heart thrives upon.

Effective exercise means the type of exercise that offers the maximum health benefit with the minimum risk of injury. One should aim for exercise that is intensive enough to keep the metabolism fast for longer periods of time and stimulate the life boosting and rejuvenating hormones - testosterone and the growth hormone. Daily engagement in exercise is necessary to keep our blood circulation, heart strength and metabolic efficiency at optimal levels. Resistance (weight) training is definitely the best method to meet these needs.

Obesity

Obesity is yet another consequence of a poor lifestyle that includes an improper diet and lack of exercise. Inactivity and a diet rich in sugars and saturated fats, whilst low in protein, fibre and essential micronutrients, causes a slow-down of our basic metabolism, an increase in body fat, a change in body composition and an increase in overall body weight. All of these ultimately lead to the condition known as obesity. Not only does obesity increase the visible body fat, it also increases the fat that surrounds internal organs. Obesity results in a total change of body composition, over-stressed vital organs such as the heart, kidneys, liver, increased stress on the joints and improper hormonal balance.

A slow metabolism (a physiologically inefficient sum of chemical processes related to the metabolism of sugar) can only be sped up and made more efficient by an increase in the tissues that burn the most energy (skeletal muscles) and by consuming foods that require more energy to be digested. Yet again we arrive at the one and only solution to tackling obesity: healthy eating and effective exercise! Obesity greatly increases the risk of cardiovascular diseases, cancer, and diabetes. It is definitely the quiet winner among the major causes of deadly disease in modern civilisation. The availability of so many kinds of food and its low cost, coupled with a lack of motivation, depression, modern trends, lack of exercise and, most importantly, lack of information about the food/health connection, have all led to an unprecedented worldwide increase in obesity.

Although the reasons that can drive a person to become obese are vast, a lack of knowledge about healthy eating and effective exercise should be considered as the major cause. Regardless of what can lower one's motivation to stay fit and healthy, it is only possible to get fat by over-eating and remaining physically inactive. Creating extra body fat and becoming overweight is only possible by over-consuming calories on a daily basis and creating a surplus that is stored as body fat. This ultimately means eating too much and the wrong kind of food! By doing so, one ingests more calories than are burned on a daily basis and the body will have to store this in the form of body fat. This is the mechanism by which one becomes fat. It is impossible to get fat in any other way. Unfortunately, the medical establishment still blindly believes in and uses body mass index as the only measurement of the "correct" body weight, undermining the fact that metabolically, the most efficient tissues regarding obesity are skeletal muscles. Skeletal muscles are heavy, and if there are more of them (bigger muscles), it automatically leads to a faster metabolism. However, with more muscle mass it is still possible to end up in the red part of the body mass index chart, qualifying as obese! Instead of using body composition (the proportion of skeletal muscles to body fat) as the ultimate guideline in suggesting a healthy weight and eliminating the risk of obesity, doctors are still relying on the completely irrelevant body mass index, which misinforms and sends the wrong message to the public.

The correct information - about natural foods, their superiority over artificial foods, the importance of eating foods rich in essential components at regular intervals and keeping active on a daily basis in order to stimulate and keep metabolism efficient - is of the utmost importance in order to maintain a healthy body weight and prevent obesity. As we have seen, so-called chronic diseases such as high blood pressure, high cholesterol levels, diabetes and heart disease are actually not diseases. They are all consequences of over-production of a single hormone in the body, insulin, due to the wrong diet. Once we force the pancreas to over-produce insulin for a certain period of time, we can expect our health to deteriorate in many ways.

The way in which one's body responds to an abnormal presence of insulin depends on one's genetic make-up. Some people develop high blood pressure, some respond with insulin resistance and others react however their genetics dictate. The bottom line is that, once the fine balance between the hormones responsible for sugar metabolism (glucagons and insulin) is disturbed, there is a definite possibility of the development of serious health consequences (which have been wrongly identified as chronic diseases). Once identified, all these conditions are treated as diseases and not the consequences of a single major disease: the hyper-production of insulin. Treating consequences and controlling them with an arsenal of medications only serves to keep the conditions alive and only deals with the body's response to those conditions.

Once the medical establishment reconsiders its fundamental strategy in the treatment of these deadly conditions, there will be a total shift of interest from symptoms towards the actual major causes: improper lifestyle and poor diet. The foods which cause over-production of insulin will be finally blamed for all this health misfortune and treated differently. These foods should all be labelled as hazardous and eventually eliminated from the market completely.

Being much more than just the sum of different macronutrients, healthy food is perfectly balanced by nature with the correct selection, amounts, and proportions of macronutrients, micronutrients, fibre and water. As such healthy, wholesome food doesn't just bring goodness to the body; it also causes a perfect hormonal response, which is necessary for the body's proper metabolism of all essential nutrients. Perfect hormonal balance and metabolism as a result of healthy eating is the foundation of good health.

Fake "foods", stripped of their natural components like fibre, water, vitamins, minerals, and macronutrients (due to modern food production technology) are the worst choices regarding our health. These denatured edibles contain only calories and additives, sweeteners, colourings, salt, sugar, flavourings and other chemicals in order to make them tastier and have a longer shelf life. They are truly poison

for the body. In order to be digested and absorbed, these edibles take
a lot of vitamins and minerals from the body that should be left for
more important jobs. Ultimately these products weaken the immune
system and lower our energy levels. Additionally, the body has to
produce a huge number of enzymes in order to break down all the
components of these denatured products and digest them. Whilst
man-made, calorie-dense products such as bread, pasta, sweets,
cakes, etc. have no enzymes, natural food is full of them. Enzyme-
rich foods are much easier to digest; they don't stress the digestive
system or the body as a whole. No wonder that we always need
to rest after a heavy meal full of denatured food. Eating that way
causes our bodies to instantly become weaker. We feel tired and
the first thing we want to do after that kind of a meal is lay down!
Sound familiar?

The bottom line

- Humans have adapted perfectly to the food that was around them
  for most of their evolution.
- During that period, chronic diseases were unknown to humans.
- With the introduction of grains into our diet (some 10 000 years
  ago), chronic diseases first entered our lives.
- As much as they are a collective responsible, chronic diseases are
  also an individual responsibility and in the majority of cases are
  self–inflicted.
- Modern medicine has perfected methods of dealing with the
  consequences of chronic diseases, but so far little has been done
  to eliminate their causes, which explains why they are constantly
  on the rise.

- A lifestyle that includes healthy eating and effective regular exercise is the best way to prevent chronic diseases.
- Although considered to be chronic diseases by medical science, conditions such as high blood pressure, high cholesterol levels (LDL) and diabetes are actually the consequences of one single major cause: hyperproduction of insulin.
- All of the consequences of hyperproduction of insulin are preconditions for various heart problems.

Protein

Macronutrients

Macronutrients are the food components which have caloric value and that represent, together with water and fibre, the bulk of all food. The macronutrients are protein, fat and carbohydrates. All of them provide energy to the body and can be used as the energy source that we constantly need for our everyday life functions such as breathing, digestion, heartbeat, walking, exercising, etc. They can also all provide adequate energy for life. Only one of them, protein, can be used as a building material necessary for the recovery and rebuilding of essential organs, tissues, bones, nerves, blood, enzymes, and connective tissues. It's no wonder that protein's name derives from the Greek word *proteios*, meaning first, most important, and essential.

We all need a certain amount of calories every day to satisfy the basic needs of our metabolism: to have enough energy and building materials to sustain life. Macronutrients must be balanced properly in order to give us enough energy and stimulate positive hormonal balance, which yields good health. If we ingest more energy than we need for daily metabolic purposes (including energy needed for different physical activities), extra energy will be stored as body fat. If we take in less energy than we need, we will start losing weight from various places, such as body fat and muscle tissue. If the amount of daily-ingested energy (calories) equals the amount of energy that we burn for metabolic and other needs daily, our body weight will remain constant and we will not store extra energy in the form of body fat.

A proper combination of all three macronutrients in the daily diet is a very important part of healthy eating. No single macronutrient can be neglected, yet incorrect combinations or proportions of macro-nutrients are common in many of today's diets around the world. This imbalance creates malnutrition, since the lack of even a single macronutrient in a diet creates a chemical imbalance and a lack of essential food components that cannot be replaced. Unfortunately, most modern diets are only focused around the caloric value of food and not around balanced macronutrients. Macronutrients in natural food are never present by themselves. They always bring with them many other essential micronutrients, such as vitamins and minerals, as well as enzymes.

A combination of these essential components is extremely important for the health of every cell in our body. Macronutrients, correctly balanced and accompanied with the essential minerals, vitamins and enzymes, are the best guarantee of good health. Not just the health of our physical bodies, but also the health and strength of our intel-lectual existence depends on our biochemistry which is fuelled from healthy eating and effective exercise.

Protein

Protein is the most abundant substance in the body, aside from water. Almost all of the tissues in the body are made of protein. All internal organs such as the heart, brain, liver, and lungs are made of protein. Our blood, skin, arteries and bones are also all made of protein. Protein is such an important nutrient for the body that it has to be included in daily dietary intake, and also in every meal of the day! As mentioned earlier, because of its immense importance, protein inherited its name from the Greek word proteios, which means the first and most important component — it is essential and irreplaceable!

Amino acids are the building blocks of protein. There are 24 amino acids and 8 of these are essential. The term "essential" means we cannot produce them or synthesise them from other amino acids or substances in the body. These eight essential amino acids must be obtained from high quality protein foods. They are: valine, lysine, methionine, leucine, isoleucine, tryptophan, threonine and phenylalanine.

Not only must they be present in every meal, but they must also be present in a certain balance. The best choice of food which offers us all essential amino acids in perfect balance is protein food of animal origin. Meat, fish, poultry, eggs and dairy products are definitely the best choice for complete protein with all essential amino acids in perfect balance. In a perfect diet, these foods should be present in every meal that we have during the day.

Our body has a constant need for essential amino acids in order to repair and grow new tissue in all of its organs. If these essential amino acids are not supplied at regular intervals during the day, the body will take them from less important tissues in order to satisfy the needs of the more important ones. This is why protein deficiency first causes degradation in the muscles, skin, hair and nails. Our bodies will sacrifice the protein from these less important tissues in order to fulfil the needs of the critical internal organs. If you ever suffer from bad nails, hair or skin, the most likely cause is protein deficiency.

Daily consumption of quality proteins is the best way to preserve the strength of the skeletal muscles and therefore the strength of the connective tissues and bone density. If we agree that loss of strength is the first sign of aging, then one can also conclude that the most essential macronutrient to prevent early aging is, without any doubt, protein! Besides a loss of strength (usually due to inactivity and a low intake of protein over long periods), the most common visible signs related to protein deficiency are: wrinkled and dry skin, brittle nails, loss of hair, loss of muscle mass, and bad posture.

For most of human history the human diet was formed around the struggle to find enough food to survive the next day or beyond. In times and regions where good food was found in abundance (meat, fruits and vegetables and, later, fish), health and overall development were highly successful. As long as protein was present in its necessary amounts, the development and health of the skeleton, muscles, skin and teeth, the health of the cardiovascular system, height, and other health characteristics were quite good. With the implementation of agriculture, it became much easier to obtain the necessary daily caloric intake, which allowed for an explosion of the human population. The human race did benefit by an increase in numbers, but suffered in health due to protein deficiency and an overwhelming amount of carbohydrates which then became, and still remain, the bulk of the daily human diet.

A diet high in carbohydrates does provide enough calories, but it does not provide enough protein necessary for the healthy development of all body systems and ultimately overall health and wellbeing. Contrary to popular belief, malnutrition is not just the lack of calories (although it can also be caused by this), but may also be caused by the lack of a single macro- or micronutrient! It is possible to consume too many calories and even get fat, but still end up with a condition (or multiple conditions) caused by a lack of some essential amino acids. Skin, hair, and nail problems are usually the first signs of protein deficiency, or more precisely, complete protein deficiency. Protein that comes from animal sources is rich in essential amino acids and therefore provides all the necessary building blocks for the repair and growth of new tissue. This type of protein must be present in every meal of the day in order to satisfy the body's need to repair or develop tissues when necessary. In contrast to animal proteins, plant proteins that are found in foods like soy, rice, beans and lentils are not rich in all essential amino acids and therefore don't provide all the building materials needed daily for the basic physiological processes. These foods are also very rich in carbohydrates and they usually lead to over-consumption of calories. More importantly, food that is poor in essential proteins and amino acids will cause the body to request more of these in order to get enough of the essentials. This is usually the major cause of food cravings, and is why some fitness experts suggest that if someone craves sugars (carbohydrates) it is a clear sign that the person needs to eat more protein! Cravings more often indicate a need for essential nutrients (mainly protein) rather than just for calories!

A diet that is rich in essential amino acids (complete proteins) is the best way to prevent cravings and all the consequences that come from them — weight problems and obesity being the major ones. The human body is constantly in search of the essential tissue-building components. As they are only available through the food that we eat, a craving appears for more food when the initial food is deficient in essentials that the body needs. Searching for essential amino acids found only in animal proteins, the body craves more and more foods (which in modern diets are poor in essential amino acids) in order to obtain the necessary amounts. This simply leads to over-consumption of other macronutrients that are less relevant, carbohydrates being the most common. Over-consumption of carbohydrates (simple and complex) is the major cause of all chronic diseases. Poor foods can only offer more calories without eliminating the problem, whilst at the same time creating an entire spectrum of undesirable health consequences.

High quality protein (containing all essential amino acids) is required in specific quantities in one's daily diet. A lack of high quality protein in a daily diet cannot satisfy the constant needs of the body to repair and grow its own tissues. These processes occur constantly in our lives: old cells in our organs and tissues die, new cells are produced, hair and nails grow, the skin and liver are repaired, enzymes are produced, red and white blood cells are formed, and many other chemical changes take place. These are just a few of the non-stop metabolic changes that, among other bodily processes, depend greatly on protein in the diet.

There are many different recommendations which have been made for our daily protein requirements. Depending on the background of the "experts" giving them, these recommended amounts vary substantially. If we take into consideration the choice of food that enables us to optimise our life potentials, and consider hunger as a signal for the next meal rather than what the clock says, the amount of protein needed in our 3 - 5 meal per day regime will depend on many different factors. Gender, age, lean body weight, and the amount, intensity and frequency of physical activities are some of the more important factors which create different protein requirements in different individuals. Taking these important factors into consideration, anything between 1 and 4 grams of protein per kilogram of lean body weight per day is the correct amount of protein that one would need in their daily diet.

Protein has an energy value (as do carbohydrates and fat) and, apart from its body building properties, it can be also used as fuel by the body. Every gram of protein is worth 4 calories, so, for example, 120 grams of protein consumed in a daily diet yields 480 calories. Although relying only on caloric measurements in creating the perfect diet is the last thing we should do, knowing the caloric value of macronutrients can only help us get the most complete information about the food that we eat.

Being the most powerful tool for creating dependence (individual and collective), food has always been an important source for taxation throughout history and a powerful money making commodity for manufacturers and governments around the world. The political and economic nature of food simply cannot be taken out of the equation. Because of this the first to suffer in the political arena of the modern world is protein; protein food is expensive, and it is difficult to produce enough of it. Consequently protein cannot be promoted and advocated as heavily as carbohydrates, which are cheap and produced around the world in quantities that even surpass the western world's demand!

It's no wonder that millions of tonnes of grains are destroyed every year, or transformed into so-called "friendly fuels"! The reason for this political practice is the preservation of the price of foods such as grains, foods that are one of the most important commodities available in the world's markets. If such massive quantities of any substance are produced, it then becomes necessary to sell in quantity, and therefore markets must be created for the product. If such large quantities of grain are produced, then it becomes necessary to find as many mouths as possible to eat that food! All the glory, marketing and justification efforts go to carbohydrates, because they absolutely need it! Biologically inferior foods have received the attention of the masses whilst the same masses have paid the heavy price attached to them. They have paid, and are still paying, with their health.

We can understand the political nature of food, but our bodies cannot. The human body still needs premium components to grow, reproduce, recover and rebuild itself; the premium component in food has always been and still is protein, the molecular backbone of every tissue in the body.

The bottom line

- Protein is the most important macronutrient and is necessary for the growth and repair of all tissues in the body.
- 8 of the 22 amino acids are essential (the human body cannot produce them) and they must be obtained from protein-rich food on a daily basis.
- Protein-rich food is rarely overeaten. Food which contains low amounts of protein or low quality protein is often overeaten simply because the body needs more of it in order to satisfy its high protein demand.
- Carbohydrate sources (foods) contain low quality protein.

Fat

Fat is another crucial macronutrient and has great importance in a healthy diet. Contrary to the popular beliefs that fat is the worst component of food, and that only food low in fat can be considered healthy and eaten safely, fat is essentially important to our health and is necessary for optimal metabolic functioning. The food that we eat should contain fat, but it must be of the right type and present in the right amounts.

Foods that have been stripped of their natural fat content (low-fat products) are not the best choices for us and are actually detrimental to our health in many cases. The fact that more low-fat products are eaten today than ever before, and that at the same time we suffer more from chronic disease than ever before, illustrates the modern fat paradox. While eating all these fat-free foods we are getting fatter and obese like never before! Almost every food available today has its low-fat variation: low-fat meats, low-fat sausages, low-fat cheese, low-fat milk, low-fat yoghurt, low-fat bread, low-fat cookies, low-fat ice cream and many others. People are becoming paranoid about consuming food that is not extremely low in fat, whilst forgetting to look at the other macronutrients in those same low-fat products which often have high caloric value. One would think that by eating more of these low-fat foods we would definitely become leaner and healthier as a nation. In reality the situation is completely opposite: low-fat foods haven't made us healthier and leaner, they have made us fatter and more prone to chronic diseases.

In order to understand the importance of fat in daily diets we will have to first understand the different types of fat and what functions they serve in the human body.

There are two major groups of fat: saturated and unsaturated. The difference between these two types lies in their ability to link with other substances in the body. Fat is composed of carbon atoms. Every carbon atom has one or more free bonds available to link with other atoms. Saturated fats have already used up all of their bonds and are linked with other substances, whereas unsaturated fats still have one or more free bonds available.

Unsaturated Fats

Unsaturated and saturated fats also have different dynamics. Unsaturated fats are more active in the body, transporting important elements such as vitamins and other nutrients, and also help to build the cell membranes all around the body. The body can also easily turn them into energy for its various metabolic requirements.

All unsaturated fats have the ability to protect cells from mutation, which is important in cancer protection. Saturated fats have no such ability. Unsaturated fats are also easier for the body to process, so they can be easily used for energy instead of being deposited throughout the body as fat. Because of this they are always the better choice when it comes to overall health and fitness. Changing the regular intake of saturated fats in one's everyday diet to unsaturated fats has a great impact on one's health.

Unsaturated fats can be further split in two groups: monounsaturated and polyunsaturated. Monounsaturated fats have one free
bond available. They are found, for example, in olive oil, almonds,
and macadamia nuts. The most important monounsaturated fat is
called oleic acid and it plays an important role in keeping our arteries supple and helping with cell membrane development and cell
formation. Monounsaturated fats are also known to lower the level
of "bad" LDL cholesterol and increase the level of "good" HDL
cholesterol, greatly improving the balance between these two types
of cholesterols.

Polyunsaturated fats are those fats whose fatty acids have more than
one free bond available to link with other nutrients. Essential fatty
acids (EFA) belong in this group and are essential for our health
simply because they cannot be synthesized by the body, and therefore have to be obtained from food sources that are rich in them.
Essential fatty acids (EFA) have to be obtained through the diet
regularly, otherwise unwanted health consequences will occur. The
two essential fatty acids are linoleic acid (LA) and alfa-linolenic
acid (NLA).

Lack of essential fatty acids in today's diet is very common. Low-fat
diets are a major health risk to people who follow them. There is a
whole chain of unhealthy reactions in the body caused by deficiency
of LA and NLA in one's daily diet. These are just a few of them:

- Heart and circulatory problems
- Skin problems
- Liver problems
- Kidney problems
- Loss of hearing

- Weakened immunity
- Weakness
- Behavioural changes
- High triglyceride levels
- High blood pressure
- Edema
- Dry skin
- Low metabolic rate

Many essential chemical processes in the body are supported by the involvement of essential fatty acids. EFA are involved in the body in producing energy from the food that we eat. They are very much involved in the oxidation processes, and therefore in energy transport EFA are also involved in oxygen transport at the molecular level, that is, transporting oxygen through the cell membranes into the cells. Essential fatty acids are also components of all cell membranes, whose health and efficiency directly depend on EFA presence. EFA are also the precursors of prostaglandins, hormone-like substances responsible for many vital processes that maintain the health of various bodily systems, especially the cardiovascular system. All of these important functions that EFA support and control in our body illustrate the great importance of EFA for our overall health. The best sources of EFA are flax oil, safflower oil, hemp seed oil and green leafy vegetables.

There are also two very important polyunsaturated fats: omega-3 and omega-6 fatty acids. Omega-3 fatty acids are found in oily ocean fish such as mackerel, sardines, herring, tuna (fresh) and salmon. Omega-6 fatty acids are found in vegetable oils such as corn oil, safflower oil and sunflower oil. The right balance between omega-3 and omega-6 is very important to our health. From our modern diets we obtain more than enough omega-6 fatty acids; however we often lack enough omega-3 fatty acids. By eating fish that is rich in omega-3 more often (3-6 times per week), or simply supplementing our diet with fish oil or cod liver oil (which are both rich in omega-3), we can dramatically improve the balance between the two and thereby enhance our health.

The benefits of omega-3 in the body are great and have been well proven throughout human history. During the times when most of our diet consisted of animal food (lean meats and fish), and in the cultures that relied mainly on fish and meat in their diets, there was always a high presence of omega-3. In those times and cultures, chronic diseases didn't exist and people tended to be much leaner, taller and healthier in general.

There are two long-chain omega-3 acids in particular that are of primary importance to our health; eicosapentaenoic acid (EPA) and docosahexaenoic acid (DHA). Through direct involvement in controlling the production and balance of some of the most important hormones (eicosanoids: autocrine hormones), EPA maintains the health of the cardiovascular system, prevents strokes, heart attacks, hypertension, arthritis, cancer, chronic infections, depression, reduces pain, enhances the immune system and more. DHA is responsible for healthy brain functioning and can stimulate growth of the nerve cells.

The recommended dose of fish oil is between 3 to 8 grams per day depending on lean body size, physical activity, age and gender. This amount of fish oil is enough to keep one's omega-3 and omega-6 in healthy balance which provides the best chance of good health.

Saturated Fats

Saturated fats are the fats that have no free bonds available to link with other molecules in the body. They are metabolically inferior to the unsaturated oils that are integral to many essential processes in the body, and they are the simplest fat found in food.

Saturated fats are found mainly in animal products such as fatty meats, lard, butter, hard cheese, cream, and also in coconut and palm oil, but are also present in smaller amounts in other oils. Over-consumption of saturated oils has been connected with arteriosclerosis and cardio-vascular diseases. They especially pose health risks when continu-ously eaten in combination with sugars and refined carbohydrates. Processed edibles like pastries, cakes and biscuits are very high in saturated fats and fast carbohydrates, and should be avoided com-pletely. Saturated fats are more difficult for the body to metabolise into heat (energy) and are more likely to end up stored as fat tissue.

Cholesterol

A few words must also be said about cholesterol. As previously mentioned, it is a waxy fat-like substance that occurs naturally in all our tissues, especially in the cell membranes. Cholesterol has al-ways been associated with poor cardiovascular health and is still the most feared substance in food. This fear has driven many people to completely eliminate cholesterol from their diets and stick to a very low-fat diet. However, cholesterol is essential for many processes in the body. Cholesterol is so essential that every cell in the body produces it. In response to dietary cholesterol, our body produces more or less of it every day. Cholesterol is essential for maintaining the fluidity of cell membranes and especially of the cells in the liver, adrenal glands, skin, arteries, testes and intestines. Our body also makes steroid hormones like oestrogen, progesterone and testosterone from cholesterol. Vitamin D is also made from cholesterol. These are just some of the essential and important roles that cholesterol plays in our health.

Cholesterol cannot be dissolved in the blood and is transported through the blood stream together with lipoproteins. There are two types of these; LDL (Low Density Lipoprotein), known as "bad cholesterol"; and HDL (High Density Lipoprotein), known as "good cholesterol". LDL is often found in arterial cholesterol deposits, while HDL has the opposite effect and cleans these deposits from the arteries. As long as they are in healthy balance, HDL and LDL function in the body without harmful effects. Foods high in sugar, refined carbohydrates, or hydrogenated oil, as well as over-consumption of alcohol, stress and inactivity, all contribute to higher levels of LDL in the blood and therefore create a higher risk of cardiovascular disease.

Foods rich in EFA (essential fatty acids), unrefined natural food, plenty of vegetables and fruit in the daily diet, relatively low carbohydrate intake and enough complete proteins, coupled with regular exercise, are the best regulators of a healthy balance between HDL and LDL in the body which promotes good cardiovascular health.

Hydrogenated Fats

Hydrogenated fats must be mentioned due to their widespread presence in everyday food and their devastating effect on our health.

Hydrogenated fat is produced by forcing hydrogen gas through vegetable oil. Products manufactured from hydrogenated fat tend to last longer without going bad and are also solid at room temperature. Although made from vegetable oils that are composed of unsaturated fats, hydrogenated fat contains saturated fats due to the process of hydrogenation.

Products made from hydrogenated fats include margarine, shortenings, shortening oils and partially hydrogenated vegetable oils. These products are widely used in chocolate, biscuits, cakes and similar foods that contain solid fats at room temperature.

Hydrogenated fats contain high levels of trans-fatty acids which are known to increase cholesterol, disrupt the functions of EFA, increase the chance for arteriosclerosis, lower immunity, increase blood insulin, and increase the chance of developing some forms of cancer.

Hydrogenated fats and the products made from them should be considered harmful to our health and avoided as much as possible. Vegetables and fruit, lean protein sources and healthy oils can help us eliminate any exposure to hydrogenated fats.

With the information learned in this chapter, we should be motivated to make our diets healthier. Fast food and diets high in saturated and hydrogenated fats cause many health problems around the world. Low-fat or fat-free diets are not much healthier, causing deficiency in essential fatty acids and thereby preventing the body from achieving optimal health. Diets that optimize our health contain lean sources of protein, especially fish rich with omega-3 fatty acids, lots of fresh vegetables, fruit, and can be supplemented with healthy oils (flax oil and others) and all essential vitamins, minerals and trace elements.

Knowing about healthy eating is the first step towards motivating yourself to eat more healthily, which is the final stage in the process. So now that you know what you have to do, make an effort and treat yourself to the best possible food choices!

The bottom line

- Bad health, associated with high-fat diets, has driven people towards low-fat or fat-free products.
- Despite this, since the introduction of low-fat and fat-free products we have witnessed an increase in obesity and chronic disease.
- Eliminating fat completely from the diet is unhealthy.
- There are two major types of fat: unsaturated and saturated.
- Unsaturated fat can be further split into two groups: monounsaturated and polyunsaturated.
- Two essential fatty acids (the human body cannot manufacture them) belong to the group of polyunsaturated fats. They are linoleic acid (LA) and alfa linolenic acid (LNA).
- The best sources of essential fatty acids are flax oil, safflower oil, hemp oil and green leafy vegetables.
- Two more very important fatty acids are omega-3 fatty acid and omega-6 fatty acid. Omega-3 fatty acid is less present in everyday food in general and it needs to be taken in higher amounts. The best natural sources are ocean fish such as herring, mackerel, salmon, sardines and tuna. Omega-3 fatty acids can also be supplemented in the form of fish oil.

Carbohydrates

The main purpose of carbohydrates in our diet is to provide energy. Unlike proteins and essential fats, which provide essential building materials for our cell membranes, nerves, blood cells, skin, internal organs, muscles etc., carbohydrates have a single purpose: to provide energy for the metabolic processes in the body. They are not involved in the growth, repair, or maintenance of tissues and organs in the body. There are no essential carbohydrates! Basically, there is no physiological requirement for carbohydrates as there is for proteins and fats.

Carbohydrates (glucose or blood sugar) can be synthesized by the body out of existing proteins and fats, and don't have to be present in our daily diets for the normal functioning of the body. Increasingly, research is showing that the fewer carbohydrates we have in our daily diet, the better health and leaner shape we will achieve. Before we get into daily requirements of carbohydrates, we need to understand their history and the different types available. We also have to learn about glycemic index and glycemic load, and our hormonal response to carbohydrates and their role in promoting obesity and chronic diseases.

Carbohydrates represent the bulk of a typical modern diet. Most of the calories that we eat on a daily basis come from carbohydrates. They began dominating the human diet some 10 000 ago and are still the most common, most preferred and most advocated source of calories in modern diets. Although we have been exposed to carbohydrate dominance in everyday diets for approximately 10 000 years we have yet to adapt to this situation. Thanks to carbohydrate dominance in our diets, humans are now suffering from a string of chronic diseases that didn't exist before the discovery of agriculture.

In the Palaeolithic period, some 10 000 to 40 000 years ago when we developed into the human form and shape that we know now, the diet of our ancestors was very different from our diet today. To start with, they didn't eat grains (which didn't exist back then) and their diet was composed predominantly of meat and — in the regions where the climate allowed — fruit and vegetables. If you bear in mind that the ability to store food for later use (freezing, cooking, packing, etc.) was non-existent, they were restricted to eating whatever was available seasonally. Since fruits and vegetables are generally available for 3-4 months per year, the only food that they could rely on year-round was meat in the form of small lizards, snails, small game, shellfish, and, later, fish and bigger animals.

The food that made us human consisted of up to 70% animal and 30% plant in origin. Carbohydrates from fruits and vegetables never represented more than 35% of the human diet. It is very important to understand that those carbohydrates in fruits and vegetables were always consumed in conjunction with an abundance of minerals, vitamins, enzymes and fibres which are found in those types of food. They were never isolated from other essential ingredients, as they are in modern diets in the form of processed food. When eaten in such a natural combination with vitamins, minerals, enzymes and fibre, carbohydrates are properly assimilated by our bodies, without a huge surge of insulin. With all the minerals, vitamins and fibre present in fresh fruits and vegetables, carbohydrates from these foods came with a rather low glycemic index. All these factors (food structure and composition) have caused our bodily systems to evolve and respond perfectly to this type of food, granting people strong immunity and lives free of chronic diseases. Palaeolithic people were also taller, stronger and much leaner than people of our time. These lessons from the past cannot be ignored.

As we have only been exposed to the dominance of carbohydrates in the last 10 000 years (a very short period in terms of our evolution), we still haven't adapted to them and cannot respond to a high carbohydrate diet without suffering from ill-health effects. As soon as they enter our mouth, carbohydrates in any form start penetrating our enamel and prepare the ground for tooth decay. A simple visit to the Egyptian section of the British Museum provides great insight for all those who still believe that carbohydrates are our best choice as a staple food. Advocates of high carbohydrate diets need only see the teeth of the mummies – who, by the way, died at very early ages (usually in their twenties) from cardiovascular diseases. The few remaining teeth in the jaws of almost all the mummies (most have been lost due to extensive carbohydrate diets) are decayed and black. And those guys didn't even eat sugar and sweets like we do today. Their main source of carbohydrates was bread which, although made up of complex carbohydrates and not white flour, converts into much simpler sugars in the mouth which are as deadly as the white sugar we are exposed to today.

In the rest of the digestive system, carbohydrates continue to upset the hormonal equilibrium and simply wreak havoc by provoking a surge of hormonal insulin (needed to lower the blood sugar level by transferring it to the energy storage points in the body). Confusion arises when we come to this point; many nutritionists have attempted to defend the "importance" of carbohydrates by trying to confront two different types of carbohydrates, blaming one type and praising the other. The only problem with their consistent efforts is that, although more people started eating their favourite healthy types of carbohydrates, our health situation has since deteriorated and is not improving; in fact it is getting worse.

There are two types of carbohydrates. The first are simple carbohydrates: monosaccharides like blood sugar (glucose) and fruit sugar (fructose), and disaccharides like milk sugar (lactose) and table sugar (sucrose). Secondly come complex carbohydrates: polysaccharides, which are found in starches and fibre (cellulose). For some reason complex carbohydrates have found more advocates among modern nutritionists who believe that, because it takes longer to break down complex carbohydrates than simple ones, they are somehow much safer for our health. Moreover, because of their complexity, they have been awarded the title "healthy" carbohydrates, instantly gaining them dominance in so-called "healthy" diets where they comprise an astonishing 60-70 percent of total daily calories! And guess what? The most common question that I'm asked by people who come to me for nutritional and fitness consultations is: "I don't understand why I have become fat when I was always eating healthily - lots of complex carbohydrates, very little fat and some protein?"

Whilst, rightfully, sugar, white flour, white rice, white pasta and other refined carbohydrates/edibles are blamed for a lot of health problems, I would include all the other starches like whole grains, brown rice, brown pasta etc. right alongside them. Although unrefined complex carbohydrates have more fibre than their refined cousins, they still cause the same unwanted hormonal response by creating high blood sugar levels. The pace of their release in the blood is not as important as many nutritionists tend to believe; the most important aspect is the overall load of sugar in the blood that results from eating starches.

Throughout our evolution vegetables and fruits have been our major source of carbohydrates and our bodily systems have developed around them. If we understand that these foods contain no more than 12% carbohydrates in even the sweetest samples (pears, plums, grapes...), then one need not be a rocket scientist to explain why we suffer when we consume foods that are, on average, made up of 70% carbohydrates (grains, pasta, rice, bread - white or brown - etc.)! That is far too much sugar for our body to handle safely, and is the major reason why diets high in carbohydrates (both simple and complex) promote an increase in body fat, obesity, and chronic diseases.

Glycemic Index

For decades glycemic indexing was the most powerful weapon used by advocates of high carbohydrate and complex carbohydrate diets, who still believe this. A glycemic index indicates the speed that sugar is released into the blood after a particular food that has been eaten. The lower the glycemic index, the slower the sugar output to the blood is, and the safer that particular food is considered. The highest possible glycemic index is 100; the closest to 100 is glucose.

The lowest glycemic indexes (up to 40) belong to most fruits (except bananas and dried fruit) and vegetables (except carrots). The highest glycemic indexes (from 60 to 90) belong to white and brown sugar, honey, syrup, white flour, cereals, white pasta, white rice, sweets, cakes, etc. Brown versions of rice, bread and pasta have a slightly lower glycemic index, but are still very high. In the middle (40-60) we find food like oatmeal, rye bread, sweetcorn, sweet potato, yams, etc. The problem with glycemic index charts is that all the foods tested for their sugar release time have been tested after being eaten on their own, without additional food being consumed at the same time. It is very unlikely that, in an average meal, any of the foods mentioned above would be eaten on their own; instead, they will have been combined with some source of protein and/or fat. Extra protein and fat eaten in the same meal slow down the speed of sugar release from carbohydrate- rich food. This is one of the reasons why the glycemic index cannot be used as a strong argument in order to explain or defend any carbohydrate-rich food.

What matters is not the glycemic index of the particular food on its own, but rather the glycemic load. Glycemic load represents the sum amount of carbohydrates eaten, multiplied by its glycemic index. This paints a much more realistic picture because it brings the amount of carbohydrates eaten into consideration. Eating too many low glycemic carbohydrates (as usually happens daily) will make everyone fat, since their glycemic load will be too high. Too much of a good thing is not always a better option.

I have seen many people who were almost obese, who didn't eat many starches, but ate rather a lot of low-glycemic fruit. Because of their belief that fruit is healthy food, they would eat 2-3 kg of different fruit per day. This is a case of too much good low-glycemic food (mainly fruit sugars) which is actually enough to make them fat. On the other hand, I have known very lean people who would eat 2-3 slices of toast and a jacket potato per day, all food with a very high glycemic index, but their glycemic load was much lower than the 2-3 kg of fruit per day in the other example.

The bottom line: even the "good" carbohydrates, in higher amounts than needed, will spill over their daily metabolic requirement and end up as fat. The body can only burn and safely store (in glycogen depots) certain amounts of carbohydrates daily; anything leftover will end up stored as body fat.

Here is a list of examples showing the glycemic index of various different foods. The higher the index, the more likely it is that the carbohydrates from the particular food will enter the bloodstream, quickly causing the huge surge in insulin.

Glycemic Index

Glucose	100
Potato	98
Parsnips	97
Carrots	92
Honey	87
Corn Flakes	80
Instant Potato	80
Bread (whole wheat)	72
Rice (white)	69
Bread (white)	69
Candy bar (Mars)	68
Shredded Wheat cereals	67
Rice (brown)	66
Raisins	64
Beets	64
Bananas	62
Sucrose (table sugar)	59
Sweet Corn	59

Buckwheat	54
Yams	51
All-bran cereals	51
Pasta	50
Oatmeal	49
Sweet potato	48
Orange Juice	46
Grapes	45
Whole-grain rye bread	42
Pasta (whole wheat)	42
Oranges	40
Baked beans	40
Apples	39
Yoghurt	36
Ice Cream	36
Lima Beans	36
Chick Peas	36
Milk (whole)	34
Pears	34
Milk (skim)	32
Navy Beans	31
Kidney Beans	29
Lentils	29
Peaches	29
Grapefruit	26
Plums	25
Cherries	23
Fructose	20

Now let's look at the hormonal reactions in the body after ingesting carbohydrates. It's not just that over-consumption of carbohydrates introduces a lot of excessive calories in the body, but it also creates unwanted hormonal responses. Once released into the blood, blood sugar (glucose) requires the hormone insulin to carry it through the blood. The role of insulin is to take whatever extra amount of glucose is in the blood and remove it. The higher the glucose rises above the normal level, the higher the output of insulin. Although it may seem that everything is in order and taken care of with enough insulin output, conditions in the body are not at all favourable in the presence of high insulin levels.

Insulin removes extra glucose in the blood by moving it to other parts of the body in two main ways: it stores glucose in glycogen depots in the liver and muscles, and it stores it in body fat. Many nutritionists favour the first role of insulin, while at the same time underestimating the role that it has played in presenting humans with so much grief through increased weight and obesity problems. Insulin will always transport the glucose to the glycogen stores simply because, meta-bolically, these are more important. Depleted glycogen stores cause weakness, tiredness, and will limit our physical ability to perform. However, problems arise due to a lack of understanding of the nature of glycogen storage. As I have personally experienced glycogen depletion and know how "easy" it is to deplete glycogen stores, I can freely say that the majority of people will never have problems caused by depleted glycogen stores. Trying to deplete my glycogen stores through high intensity training and a zero carbohydrate diet, in order to achieve glycogen super-reloading in the 2-3 days before a body-building competition, I have tried many times to get to the stage where all my glycogen stores were heavily depleted. I have monitored the success of these attempts by controlling urinary ketone levels. Once glycogen stores are depleted, the body starts running predominantly on fat reserves, releasing ketone bodies (by-products of fat metabolism used for energy purposes) into the urine. It would take me 4-5 days before I would enter ketosis (elevated levels of ketone bodies in the blood) to the point that would suggest my glycogen stores were quite depleted. Now just to remind you, I would train twice per day with weights — up to 1.5 hours each session — while eating only protein food that, in theory, wouldn't cause glycogen replenishment. So now, compare that with the average person who never does any weight training and never eats a diet consisting only of protein! Do you think that that person (representing the majority of people in society) would have their glycogen stores depleted, or even slightly disturbed? The answer is no; the glycogen stores will be mostly full at all times. This simply means that insulin will have to perform very little glycogen replacement management, and will drive most of the extra glucose found in the blood straight to fat deposits (i.e. body fat).

Once this has been clarified and the major role of insulin understood as controlling glucose storage in the body fat, it wouldn't be hard to understand the importance of normal insulin levels in the blood. But keeping the insulin level normal is not only important for the purpose of staying lean, it is even more important for all the other health benefits that simply disappear when there is a high presence of insulin in the blood.

The best sources of carbohydrates are vegetables and fruits. Both of them are predominantly made up of water and fibre, so they are not carbohydrate-dense like grains and grain products. Because of this it is very difficult to overeat these types of food. Vegetables consist of no more than 5% carbohydrates, while fruit consists of up to 12% carbohydrates. This is the simple reason why it is almost impossible to overeat fruit. 2-3 pieces of fruit and 3-5 portions of vegetables daily will satisfy the carbohydrate demands of even highly active people. The occasional bowl of porridge, a sweet potato, or a couple of pieces of whole grain bread wouldn't cause a problem, especially for physically active people. But making starches a staple food, as advised by so many nutritionists, leads directly to the health situation we are in right now.

The majority of people will respond to a diet high in carbohydrates (complex or simple) with a correspondingly high production of insulin, body fat build up, increased cholesterol level (high LDL), high blood pressure, higher risk of cardiovascular diseases, higher risk of diabetic development, obesity, and many other adverse reactions. Whilst glycemic indexing has won attention and tabloid headlines, and health and fitness magazines have been wrongly delivering the message about the amount and types of carbohydrates that should be eaten in order to preserve good health and burn extra body fat. Glycemic load, which is more important and has much more responsibility for overall fat accumulation or loss, has been heavily underestimated.

Glycemic Load

So what is the glycemic load? As mentioned earlier, glycemic load is the overall amount of carbohydrates eaten in the same meal, multiplied by their glycemic index. If, for example, you have 25 grams of carbohydrates with a glycemic index of 60, we multiply the weight by the glycemic index which gives us the glycemic load. 25 x 60 is 1500, meaning that the glycemic load of that particular meal would be 1500.

Now let's take a look at the meal with a glycemic index of 40, which is lower than in the previous meal at 60, and thus seems better on first glance. But if the amount of carbohydrates with the glycemic index of 40 is 120 grams, when you multiply 120 by 40 that would give us a glycemic load for this meal of 4800. Compared to the meal above, that would be 4800 vs. 1500, or more than 3 times the load! What does that mean? It means that the body would have to deal with a much larger amount of carbohydrates in a single meal, and in the process digest it into glucose and soon after metabolise it into glycogen stores or fat deposits. The outcome of consuming a higher glycemic load is a higher production of insulin due to the higher amount of glucose and a higher deposition of the same glucose into body fat.

So, the overall amount of carbohydrates we eat is of much more importance than is simply shown by their glycemic index. You can eat fewer carbohydrates with a higher glycemic index, and end up leaner than if you were to eat higher amounts of carbohydrates with a lower glycemic index.

In order to stay in good health, limit your carbohydrate sources to vegetables and fruits, with an occasional treat of a relatively low glycemic food like oatmeal, sweet potatoes or wholegrain bread. Be sure to eat a lot of lean protein foods, and include enough good fats (cold water ocean fish oil, flaxseed oil, olive oil) in your diet. Avoid products made of sugar, flour and saturated/hydrogenated fats such as chocolate, biscuits, cakes, sweets, ice cream, white and brown bread, white and brown rice, pastas, pizzas, pastries, potatoes, etc.

The bottom line

- The only role of carbohydrates in the body is to provide energy necessary for the different metabolic processes. Carbohydrates are not involved in the growth and repair of the body's tissues.
- There are no essential carbohydrates as there are essential amino acids and fatty acids; therefore we do not have a physiological need for carbohydrates.
- Glucose (blood sugar) can be manufactured from any macronutrient (protein, fat or carbohydrates).
- In evolutionary terms, carbohydrates have never accounted for more than 30 percent or our diet. Since the introduction of grains they have reached a staggering 70 percent of our diet.
- Natural carbohydrate sources like fruits and vegetables contain no more than 12 percent, while carbohydrates in grains and edibles made from grains reach up to 70 percent. Food with that high a percentage of carbohydrates causes huge surges of insulin in the body, often with bad consequences for our health.
- Regardless of whether carbohydrates are simple or complex, they both need insulin to be stored in different tissues in the body. Being "white" or "brown" doesn't make a difference in terms of insulin reaction because different grain products require the same amount of insulin due to containing the same amount of carbohydrates.
- Glycemic load is more important than glycemic index. It represents the total amount of ingested carbohydrates multiplied by their glycemic index. The lower the glycemic load, the better it is for overall health.

Sugar

I have decided to devote a whole chapter of this book to the issue of sugar — or, more precisely, refined carbohydrates. Sugar has established its presence in the human diet, and especially in the modern diet where it dominates every single meal of the day! Sugar is an unavoidable "tenant" in every single household, either in the form of table sugar, or as a component of sweets, chocolates, cakes, bread, or the many other sweetened foods and drinks commonly found in our homes. Not every one of us has tomatoes, green peppers and lettuce in the house at any given time, yet sugar and other edibles containing sugar almost certainly have a presence in every household at all times! Do you have white or brown sugar in the house right now, or biscuits, chocolate, ketchup or white bread? Of course you must have some of them. But how many of you have pears, apples, celery or cucumbers in the house right now? I bet not many. With the invasion of sugar in our diets we have also changed our criteria for healthy eating and our shopping habits, and have started consuming higher than ever amounts of calories while at the same time becoming slaves of sweetness. By believing that satisfying the urge for sweet foods can provide the ultimate comfort and help us to relax and feel better, we have actually caused a lot of ill health, misery and even death.

After a "great" meal, the common practice is to have something sweet, like ice cream, chocolate, or cheesecake. The reason: our taste for sweetness has to be satisfied, and that is the final step in the ceremony of eating! When the child does something good the reward is usually a biscuit or chocolate. Definitely not a carrot or a plum! Sugar is without a doubt the ultimate reward. And this is how most of us are trained from a very early age (baby foods are full of sugar), to identify sugar and the simulated taste of sweetness with calmness, reward, and pleasure.

After easily winning the competition for most satisfying taste, sugar has moved into other edibles to make them more enjoyable, popular and easy to sell. This is why most bread loaves, bagels or croissants you buy every day contain sugar! Breakfast cereals, most ready-made meals, fruit yoghurts and fruit juices are full of sugar; does this sound familiar to you? Sugar has been put into most processed foods in order to make them "tastier" and also better sellers. Can you recall a single day in recent times that you didn't have something sweet to eat?

Sugar is pumped into different products in such huge amounts that it regularly accounts for up to 50% of that particular product! Chocolates, biscuits, jams, sweets and cakes sometimes consist of more than 50% sugar. Now, just for the sake of sanity, compare those same products with the sugar content of naturally sweet foods (like fruits) which are no more than 12% sugar (mainly fructose). What nature has created, in order to attract us by stimulating our taste for sweetness, we have corrected by creating edibles that consist of more than 50% sugar.

Not only is it that the type of sugar we have chosen to integrate into our new foods is different than the natural sugar in fruits (white or brown table sugar has a glycemic index 4 times higher than fructose, the natural sugar found in fruit), but also that the amount of our new refined sugar is more than 4 times higher than the amount in fruits!

The gastronomy of nature is losing the battle against the gastronomy of humans! But the story of our adventures in the realm of food hasn't had a happy ending...

We have suffered badly since parting ways with the natural concepts of nutrition. New life and experiences surprised us in the form of chronic diseases and it seems that we are still in a state of shock, trying desperately to discover the major causes of our deteriorating health. Chronic diseases are responsible for most of the deaths in Western countries.

Technically there are a few different types of sugar, and the advocates of high carbohydrate diets have highlighted the importance of these differences in order to preserve the major ideas about carbohydrates and support the principle that tries to defend carbohydrates as the best staple food for humans. Advocates of high carbohydrate diets have developed a whole science concerning the different types of carbohydrates and their different roles in human physiology. These scenarios make white table sugar the villain, whilst some other types of sugar (all processed) are considered good for you!

The truth is that all refined carbohydrates (what I call refined sugars) have almost the same destiny in the human body when they are consumed. They are absorbed easily at a high rate, thereby causing a major hormonal upset with huge health consequences. If it weren't for our modern cosmetic preference for a slim figure, we would never bother trying to lose weight.

Losing extra body fat is much more important for human health than just getting leaner for cosmetic reasons is. Body fat is not only the amount of fat that accumulates around the waist, on the buttocks and legs, but also the amount of newly generated fat that surrounds our internal organs and muscles. Fat also gets inside the tissues and can increase its presence in the blood where, together with high levels of insulin and LDL, it becomes one of the major contributing factors to the narrowing of the arteries. As well as from the devastating direct effects that an increase in body fat has on human health, refined sugar consumption also lowers immunity, making the body more vulnerable to a whole range of additional diseases.

Refined carbohydrates like table sugar, white flour, white rice and starch were unknown to our ancestors for millions of years. For more than 99% of our evolution, nothing in the human diet has influenced hormonal reactions to the level that refined carbohydrates have in modern times. Our physiology, and hormonal, digestive and coronary systems (among others) evolved according to the food that was available to our ancestors for hundreds of millennia.

We have developed perfectly around that food, defending ourselves from infections and illnesses with strong immunity. Our life energy was perfectly split among our body systems; digestion for example didn't use most of our life energy, as it does in our modern times. Humans used to eat in order to live; they didn't live to eat, or to satisfy pleasure or boredom as we do nowadays. Food eaten throughout our evolution was full of enzymes, co-enzymes (minerals) and co-factors (vitamins). These essential components of food saved a great deal of digestion. The dry and processed foods that we indulge in today in huge amounts, robbed of their own enzymes, minerals and vitamins, are a burden to our digestive system. In order to digest food that is stripped of its own enzymes, the digestive system (stomach, liver, and pancreas) has to produce huge amounts of enzymes. This effort is what requires great amounts of life energy, leaving less of it for the immune system. Used disproportionately for digestion only, our life energy that should be available to other systems like immunity, the muscular system, the recovery system, etc., is greatly depleted. Yet we still pray for good health and regard it as a gift (or simply luck), rather than the expected outcome of a healthy lifestyle in which healthy eating plays an essential role.

Lately the government has been trying hard to deliver the message that fresh fruit and vegetables are the answer to strong immunity and good health, but at the same time they never try to explain why. Because of this, people still continue to gobble huge amounts of processed foods, or dead foods as I like to call them. The government has never explained that processed food is nothing but the empty caloric residue of natural food robbed of enzymes, fibre and micronutrients. Modern foods full of sugar and carbohydrates, such as cereals, bread, rice, pasta, sweets, cakes, pastries, juices, and many other money-making food inventions that disappear into the guts of billions of people every single day, are nothing more than a bunch of empty calories. On the other hand, natural food is full of essential nutrients. The right combination and amount of amino acids in meat and fish, and the vitamins, minerals and enzymes found in fresh fruits and vegetables, are what our body recognises and accepts with ease. The natural combination of microelements is the ideal environment for optimal absorption and contribution to enzyme production. Adding one of the micronutrients in higher or lower amounts knocks them out of their natural balance, impairing their functions.

Let's now take a look at the direct interaction that sugar has with our own biochemistry. Let's look at the body's very delicate production of enzymes and hormones, its synthesis of vitamins and minerals, and their involvement in essential chemical reactions within the human body — all of which become impaired with the aggressive over- presence of sugar.

The biggest problem we face in the presence of high amounts of re-fined sugars in the bulk of modern man's daily diet is hyper-insuline-mia, or hyperproduction of insulin (simultaneously one of the most important and most deadly hormones produced by the body). This hormone is so important that, without it, life would not be possible. At the same time however, insulin is a hormone that can literally kill you if produced in large enough amounts.

Eating refined sugars in large amounts can cause a sudden high production of insulin. Refined sugars are very easily digested, being stripped of natural fibre, enzymes, vitamins and minerals, but are also very unsatisfying foods. When you eat refined sugars you will never be satisfied with a small or even medium amount, because their physical volume is very small (no water or fibre content) and therefore more refined sugars have to be eaten in order to satisfy the ordinary hunger that appears before regular meals. This is why you will always end up eating more than the sufficient amount of refined sugars than your body can handle in a single meal. The amount of sugar that will enter the blood (blood sugar or glucose) will be higher than the body's capability to store it in the safe glycogen stores. This raised level of blood sugar is called hyperglycemia, and the hormone insulin will be needed in high amounts in order to lower the blood sugar levels and protect the brain. Most of the extra sugar from the blood will be stored in the form of body fat, while insulin will continue to lower the blood sugar levels to below their normal levels! The scenario that will occur after heightened insulin levels is one of very low blood sugar, known as hypoglycemia.

First hyperglycemia, and then hypoglycaemia; these are the problems that arise from the high consumption of refined sugars. Increased insulin production is linked to all major cardiovascular diseases such as high blood pressure, arteriosclerosis, high cholesterol levels and strokes, obesity, and other diseases. In the presence of high insulin, the condition known as hypoglycemia (low blood sugar levels) will occur, causing health problems including depression, aggression, weakness, insomnia and others. Both hyperglycemia and hypoglycemia are caused by the overeating of refined sugars. Hypoglycemia will start new cravings for sweets. By eating them a person will progress to the stage of hyperglycemia which then triggers a massive release of insulin, which in turn creates the state of hypoglycemia again. This unavoidable cycle will repeat itself as long as we engage in a diet high in carbohydrates.

When refined sugars enter the body, they are taken for nothing else other than an amount of empty calories that the body has to deal with. Refined sugars are also called empty calories because they don't bring anything else into the body with them apart from caloric (energy) value. Unlike refined sugars, natural foods contain other ingredients like enzymes, vitamins, minerals, trace elements and fibre. Refined sugars are completely devoid of all these, therefore requiring a big effort from the body to digest and assimilate them. The problems occur when the body has to give up all the necessary micronutrients so that it can metabolise the refined sugars. Once the body loses its vitamins, minerals and trace elements in this manner, it becomes less able to perform efficiently in other important areas where these micronutrients are essential, such as the metabolism of fat and cholesterol, the elimination of cholesterol from the body, and the burning of fat. Intake of refined sugars will depress the body's ability to perform the above-mentioned duties efficiently and leads to consequences such as high cholesterol levels, slower fat burning ability, slower metabolism and, of course, weight gain. Fat gain usually leads to obesity, creating conditions for lower insulin sensitivity and ultimately for diabetes. Obesity also increases the risk of developing cardiovascular disease and some forms of cancer. A whole range of other diseases also begin with weight gain and obesity.

Other damaging effects of sugar intake include a weakening of the immune system and the development of food allergies — with all their health damaging consequences like joint pain, asthma, auto-immune disease, muscle pain and more.

Lack of fibre in food containing refined sugar also slows the passage of food through the intestines. Because such foods remain in the colon too long, fermentation of the same causes gas and toxins from bad bacteria that feed on refined sugars. Constipation is easily caused by this lack of fibre and can cause many health problems, including bowel cancer.

Sugar consumption also increases the production of adrenal hormones by up to 4 times! High levels of adrenalin increase production of cholesterol in the body and also of the hormone cortisone, the catabolic hormone that inhibits immune system functions.

Refined sugars interfere with the production of collagen and elastin (through decreased transportation of vitamin C in the body), both necessary for the strength of all connective tissues, arteries, skin and other tissues. Disrupted healthy production of collagen and elastin are the major causes of premature aging and increased wrinkling of the skin.

Sugar is also the worst enemy of tooth enamel. During our early evolution, no food containing refined sugar entered the human mouth and therefore the protection of the teeth and gums from refined sugars wasn't necessary. We have no natural protection for our teeth and gums either against unnatural substances, or from sugar in the first place. Certain types of bacteria produce acid that simply drills through enamel and enables bacteria to form and multiply, culminating in caries and other tooth and gum diseases. Sugar fuels this production of bacterial acid. By regularly eating refined sugars and starches we are simply promoting acid production from bacteria, cavity formation in our teeth, and gum disease. The most explicit proof for the damaging effect of sugar on our teeth and gums is found in human remains from different stages throughout history. Pre-agricultural remains (10 000 years or older) of humans show perfect jaw development with all the teeth in their perfect size and numbers, without any caries on them. Remains of humans that date after the discovery of agriculture show a different picture; the jaw is smaller, the teeth overlap each other, and tooth decay caused by caries is always present. Gum disease is also widespread in agricultural humans, while non-existent in pre-agricultural periods. Another drastic example of the devastating effect of sugar on our teeth is the current widespread prevalence of caries and gum disease. Do you know anyone who doesn't have one or more fillings in their mouth? I don't.

Being the main villain in our diet, sugar robs the most essential microelements for its own metabolism. Just to remind you, essential vitamins and minerals are the body's biggest assets. It takes time and perfect nutrition (a quality and amount that is very difficult to obtain in a modern lifestyle) to refill the stores of essential minerals, vitamins and trace elements that are eventually lost while metabolising sugar. Losing these assets is the fastest way to weaken the body's systems.

Instead of relying on medical help in order to treat the health consequences caused by a regular intake of refined sugars, a much better solution would be to eliminate their cause in the first place. Avoid refined sugars (table sugar, white flour products, white rice, bread etc.) completely and concentrate on natural food only. The bulk of your food should be made of vegetables and different types of meat and fish, while fruit should be eaten in moderation.

The bottom line

- Sugar and refined starches make up most of the food that are regarded as staples in western societies.
- Even unknowingly, sugar and refined starches are eaten in large amounts simply because they have become ingredients in the majority of edibles.
- Being refined, these carbohydrates are stripped of all the necessary minerals, vitamins and enzymes found in natural food. In order to digest and absorb them, our body needs to sacrifice its own precious storage of those microelements.
- Intake of sugar and refined starches causes hyperglycemia (high blood sugar level), which is then followed by hypoglycemia (low blood sugar level). These two conditions can repeat back and forth daily depending on how many times sugar is eaten.
- Because humans have evolved without exposure to sugar and refined starches, we have no protection against them. They cause a whole chain of bad health reactions.

Food Intolerance and Food Allergies

Although humans have developed the great ability to eat almost anything in order to survive, that doesn't mean that eating everything will do us good in the long term. The ability to eat different types of food in certain circumstances just to survive can be beneficial to the species, but when the choice of food is large and its availability constant, we have to opt for the best food, not just any food. That means that we should strive to eat foods that do us good and that are easily digested and optimally absorbed without over-taxing the digestive system. We should be seeking foods that don't cause inflammation, unwanted chemical reactions, disrupted digestion, or limit the absorption of nutrients.

Food allergies, and especially food intolerance, have been widespread since the introduction of grains and milk into the human diet. Once they entered the diet, grains and milk began to cause many health problems, which have developed into chronic diseases previously unknown to the human species. But they also have caused immediate adverse reactions in the digestive and immune systems, signalling that humans were not, and are still not, ready to safely eat those types of food. Food intolerance and food allergies are two different physiological reactions that occur when certain types of food enter the body

While food intolerance mainly manifests itself within the digestive system with its refusal of certain foods (reactions include migraine, indigestion, bloating, gas, diarrhoea, etc.), food allergies are an immune response to certain food components. When the body recognizes certain food components (casein, gluten, etc.) as allergens or foreign invaders, the immune system reacts by sending antibodies (immunoglobulin E) to destroy the molecules of the mistakenly identified antigens. This drastic reaction of the immune system causes the production of histamine in certain tissues and consequent swelling (nose, lips, tongue, throat and gut), skin reactions such as red rashes, or in extreme cases, anaphylactic shock. Food allergies can be life threatening, but even though less widespread than food intolerance, food allergies can develop from long-term food intolerances where the body becomes overly sensitive to foods that cause such chronic intolerance.

There is one widespread phenomenon of food intolerance that has been ignored by the majority of people throughout our history. If someone gains an extra 5-10 pounds or more of extra body weight due to simple water retention, this is usually considered a normal condition. But what is not understood is that water retention is only a consequence of a deeper underlying problem caused by food intolerance, which may lead to other more serious health problems. In order to understand the major causes of food intolerance, we have to look back into the human evolutionary adaptation to living environments, whilst distinguishing between the nutritional conditions that have allowed genetic adaptation and the conditions that have appeared in relatively modern history (10 000 years ago) causing adverse physical reactions.

If you look at any other mammal species and their eating habits, you will find that none of them eat anything other than the food that has been around them for hundreds of thousands of years. Imagine an herbivore choosing meat, or a carnivore feeding on grass! We never imagine these kinds of things; we accept that every species eats the food that they are genetically geared to eating, or in other words, the food that they have evolved around. These facts apply to every single species apart from one: Homo Sapiens!

In order to avoid this anomaly, politically correct thinkers have come up with a perfect solution: use the term omnivore to cover up our wrong-doing (wrong eating)! Omnivores are the mammals that eat both plants and meat, while carnivores eat only meat and herbivores eat only plants. Nothing is wrong with that as long as we stick to the vegetables, fruits and meats that have been around us for 99% of our evolution. However, calling ourselves omnivores in order to justify the eating of grain and milk products over the last 10 000 years, or for only 1% of our evolutionary time, is simply a cover-up and is totally unacceptable. Being omnivores is one thing; eating grain and milk products is something totally different and I would never describe those two concepts using the same term! Meat, vegetables and fruits can go under the umbrella of omnivores, but grain and milk products cannot sneak through. These new foods and their Franken-stein cousins — especially refined foods that derive from grains and milk — have caused more misery than benefit to humankind.

Nowadays, we are trying to mystify the causes of chronic disease that are devastating human cultures around the world, ignoring the simple fact that we are not following our evolutionary heritage and eating the food that humans have eaten for most of the time of our existence on this planet. Most of our health misery simply didn't exist before! Our ancestors didn't suffer from chronic diseases as we suffer today. And the major difference between us and our ancestors is in the food that we eat.

Food intolerance is the most drastic proof that we have not yet adapted to some foods and that we do produce strong chemical reactions when those foods are introduced into our digestive system. The most common reactions to foods that we have not adapted to are bloating, stomach pain, gas, diarrhoea, dehydration, loss of electrolytes, constipation, build-up of toxins, water retention, etc. While most of the above symptoms are mainly related to the upsetting of our digestive system, there are more serious consequences that occur due to prolonged eating of food that is incompatible with our bodies and causes food intolerance. The build-up of plaque in the arteries, arteriosclerosis, high blood pressure, high cholesterol levels, glucose intolerance, insulin resistance, diabetes, obesity, and other conditions are directly linked to foods that are poorly tolerated by the body.

A common problem with people who have mild food intolerance is that they usually fail to recognize the problem, and continue living with the constant discomfort of bloating, water retention, increased blood pressure and other conditions. Assuming that everything is still normal, people continue living with that mild discomfort until it develops into a more serious condition. Food intolerance has to be recognised as soon as it appears, and the causes for that intolerance need to be eliminated in order to allow the body to function with optimum efficiency.

Let's have a look at the most common foods that cause food intolerance. Grains and legumes are known to cause food intolerance in many people. Milk and milk products are another food group that is known to cause a great deal of food intolerance. So, do grains and milk have anything in common? Although they are two totally different food groups, they have one major thing in common: they have not been present in our diet for approximately 99% of our evolution! Grains and milk were introduced into the human diet some 10 000 years ago and, because of this very short evolutionary period, we haven't had enough time to adapt and respond without the typical symptoms of food intolerance. We are simply not ready yet to ingest grains and milk without some consequences to our health.

Grains

So what is wrong with grains and what do they contain that causes so much damage to human health, starting with symptoms of food intolerance? To begin with, grains are made of starches. Starches are complex carbohydrates with very high caloric value. Most grains are made up of 70% complex sugars (carbohydrates)! The food that we have evolved around for most of our evolution never contained more than 12% sugar (fruits). Vegetables contain only around 3% carbohydrates.

When we eat grains, or different food made from grains, we simply allow huge amounts of starch to enter our digestive system. On top of that, the most popular starchy foods that we eat today and that have become staple foods for the majority of the population are foods with a very high glycemic index (70 or more). This suggests that most popular starchy foods, for example potatoes, rice, bread, and breakfast cereals, are assimilated very quickly, rapidly raising the blood's glucose level. This causes high insulin release and a whole chain of unwanted health-threatening reactions with hypoglycaemia, a condition caused by low blood sugar, being just one of them. Symptoms such as tiredness, headaches, low blood pressure, irritability, nervousness, lack of concentration and more are very common among the general population. In order to fix these symptoms, people opt for high carbohydrate edibles like candies, chocolates, biscuits, potatoes, cereals, bread, etc., which only repeat the process, causing the same hypoglycaemic effects again and again throughout the day. The drastic insulin production that takes place after every high carbohydrate meal also wipes out all the sugar from the bloodstream, causing the same symptoms and trapping the sufferers in a vicious cycle.

The stomach, being an exclusively acidic environment, finds it hard to digest carbohydrates. Therefore, large amounts of carbohydrates (starch from the grains) ferment in the stomach causing bloating and indigestion due to disrupted protein digestion. In a natural scenario, protein-rich foods should be eaten on their own or with vegetables that only have very small amounts of carbohydrates (most vegetables contain only around 3% carbohydrates). Compared to the high carbohydrate content of starches in grains, small amounts of carbohydrates from vegetables and fruit will not cause any problem in the stomach's acidic environment and will not disrupt protein digestion. In order to get a clear picture of the amount and concentration of starches found in grains let me just remind you that, for example, 2 kilograms of broccoli has the same amount of digestible carbohydrates as 100 grams of cereal! So, even in small amounts, starchy foods are not as innocent as they may look.

Some grains such as wheat, rye, barley and oats contain a type of protein called gluten. Gluten is actually a mixture of two proteins, gliadin and glutenin, which become sticky when mixed with water. In many people, gluten causes digestive disturbances because of a gluten intolerance. Coeliac disease is caused by gluten intolerance and is a life-long inflammatory disease of the upper small intestine. In people with gluten intolerance, gluten damages the lining of the small intestines causing inflammation, and once inflamed, the villi (finger-like projections on the small intestine) become unable to absorb nutrients and water, causing a whole range of other diseases. Apart from not being able to absorb essential nutrients and water, the lining of the small intestine stops producing the enzymes necessary for digestion of other nutrients like lactose and carbohydrates. In this situation large particles of food remain undigested in the small intestine and, through bacterial action, begin to ferment causing cramps, gas, bloating and diarrhoea. Typical symptoms of coeliac disease are weight loss, chronic diarrhoea, anaemia, weakness and fatigue.

There are other problems with grains as well. One of them is the high content of phytic acid in bran. Phytic acid is known to bind to certain macro and micronutrients and inhibit their absorption. It also inhibits the absorption of minerals such as iron and zinc, calcium and magnesium, as well as protein and starches. There are also problems with soy beans, for example, which contain potent enzyme inhibitors that block the action of trypsin and other enzymes needed for protein digestion. Eating foods containing these inhibitors can cause serious gastric distress, reduce protein digestion, and result in chronic amino acid deficiencies. Tripsin inhibitors and heamaglutinin are also growth inhibitors.

Scientists in general agree that grain and legume-based diets high in phytates contribute to widespread mineral deficiency (especially in third world countries). Although bulk minerals such as calcium, potassium and phosphorus are present in the plant foods eaten in these areas, the high phytate content in these foods (soy and grains) prevents their absorption.

Milk

Milk and milk products are probably the most popular and trusted food for a majority of cultures. We feed everyone with milk and milk products: babies, children, adults, the elderly, even our pets! Milk is one of the major ingredients in so many different dishes; we add milk to meat dishes, to grain dishes, to sauces, to soups, we put milk into coffee, tea, chocolate drinks, we make sweets and cakes out of milk and, of course, ice cream! Simply put, milk is always present in our daily diet, in one form or another.

Despite the huge popularity and wide acceptance of milk and milk products, milk is one of the foods that causes most food allergies and food intolerances. It is well known that milk causes many digestive problems and gastric discomfort including bloating, gas, diarrhoea and weakness in many people. Apart from that, milk can cause more serious health problems in people who have developed a milk allergy. Many of these people don't realise that they suffer from milk intolerance which can easily develop into more dangerous milk allergies, simply because the symptoms are not drastic. Most people do not see a problem if they retain extra water or are constantly bloated, since it is so common that it may even be considered normal. But even moderate bloating and moderate water retention can put our health at risk. Bloating and gas disrupt digestion and absorption, whilst water retention increases blood pressure and, as extra weight, puts more stress on the cardiovascular and skeletal systems.

Now let's have a closer look at the components in milk and find out which ones are responsible for milk intolerance and milk allergies. When we talk about milk we usually talk about cow's milk. It is cow's milk that we humans have transformed into one of our staple foods. We have chosen this particular type of milk to be our food day after day, since the domestication of livestock that started some 10 000 years ago.

Cow's milk is perfectly designed to support the growth and development of their own young. Their digestive system is perfectly formed to digest cow's milk and absorb all the nutrients that it holds within. The dominant protein in cow's milk, casein, is the perfect protein for the development of the huge skeleton and muscles in a young cow's body. Casein is digested easily in the intestines of their young, but this is where the story ends with cow's milk. Once they have been weaned, calves do not want to drink milk any longer! They immediately switch to grass as their next natural food choice. The only species that continues to milk cows and drink the result as adults are humans. Whilst no other species drinks the milk from any species other than their own (or as adults), we humans do.

There are two enzymes needed to break down milk, rennin and lactase. Production of both these enzymes dramatically decreases after the age of three and, after that period, we simply are not efficient at or capable of breaking down milk successfully. In the absence of these enzymes two problems develop: first, milk sugar, or lactose, cannot be digested. Lactose needs to be broken down into glucose and galactose, to become simplified into sugars that can be absorbed by the body. If undigested due to the lack of lactase, lactose will pass through the system and be attacked by bacteria in the large intestine. That causes the fermentation of glucose, which leads to other unwanted side effects. The typical symptoms of lactose intolerance are bloating, gas and diarrhoea.

The second problem is limited digestion of casein, the dominant protein in cow's milk. The content of casein in cow's milk is many times higher than the content of casein in human milk. Cows need this high proportion of casein in their milk for the development of their massive bones. In humans, coagulated casein forms large, difficult to digest curds in the stomach. The body needs huge amounts of energy in order to somehow get rid of this material, which also sticks to the lining of the intestine, reducing the absorption of many essential nutrients.

Milk allergies are caused when milk proteins, mainly casein, are not recognised by the body and are identified as antigens. As a response, the body makes antibodies that attack antigens in order to remove them from the system. Since casein is responsible for 80% of milk proteins, it is recognised as one of the major allergens found in milk. The symptoms of milk protein allergy appear as skin reactions (red itchy rash, eczema, swelling of the lips, tongue, lips and throat), stomach and intestinal reactions (abdominal pain, bloating, gas, vomiting, diarrhoea, cramps) and nose, throat and lung reactions. Milk consumption is linked with the production of mucus in the body, which is a by-product of milk digestion. Casein is also linked with thyroid problems.

Although the consequences of food intolerance and food allergies can be treated with different medications and antihistamines which stop the body from producing histamine as a consequence of the action of immunoglobulins, the best method is still to prevent them by avoiding food that causes food intolerance and allergies in the first place.

There are many other foods that can cause allergies and intolerance, but wheat and milk, being new additions to the human diet, cause most of the allergy problems. In situations when the human body cannot recognise them as natural food, it identifies them as foreign substances (antigens). And while allergies and food intolerance do represent direct reactions to these allergens, the other more serious indirect reactions, such as hormonal and cardiovascular problems, represent a much bigger risk to us. Food intolerance and allergies manifest themselves immediately and can be dealt with straight away; other health problems take time to develop to the level when consequences appear, which unfortunately is often too late to treat them.

The bottom line

- Food intolerance and food allergies have become widespread since the introduction of grains and milk into the human diet.
- Food intolerance is mainly a response of the digestive system to food that cannot be tolerated. The most common symptoms of food intolerance are bloating, gas, water retention, diarrhoea and migraines.
- Food allergies are drastic responses of the immune system to certain components of food (gluten, casein and others). Sudden production of histamine then causes swelling of different tissues such as the nose, lips, throat, tongue and others. Food allergies can be life threatening.
- Grains and milk cause the majority of food intolerances and food allergies.

Fibre

Fibre is a very important component of food and has great health benefits for us. Dietary fibre comes from fruits, vegetables and grains, whilst animal foods such as meat, poultry, fish, eggs or milk products contain no dietary fibre. People who rely mainly on processed foods don't ingest enough fibre on a daily basis, and these foods get absorbed quickly and don't provide enough bulk to stimulate bowel movement and elimination. Because of this lack of dietary fibre, processed foods cause constipation, which leads to a whole spectrum of diseases including some types of cancer.

Constipation is one of the many common problems caused by our sedentary lifestyle and poor nutrition. It is estimated that more than 14 million people in the UK alone suffer from constipation. Among the other lifestyle-related causes, a lack of dietary fibre in every-day diets is one of the biggest contributors to constipation and can cause exhaustion, tiredness, nervousness and, ultimately, a build-up of harmful toxins in the body. Constipation is also the most common cause of haemorrhoids. Straining to pass hard stools causes too much pressure on the rectum, making the veins swell and causing haemorrhoids to appear.

There are two major types of dietary fibre: soluble and insoluble. Soluble dietary fibre can dissolve in water while insoluble cannot. Humans can't digest either of these types of fibre, and both soluble and insoluble dietary fibre have great health benefits. Examples of insoluble fibre include cellulose, lignin and hemicellulose (which is partly soluble). These have the ability to absorb a lot of water, and hemicellulose can even absorb up to 8 times its own weight in water. This ability of insoluble fibre to store water is of extreme importance in promoting a large and soft stool, which then decreases the stool's passage time through the body. Regular daily stools are the best guarantee for the health of the colon and other intestines, as they keep them clean and free of unfriendly and harmful bacteria.

Soluble fibre dissolves in water. It binds with certain substances and removes them from the gut, cleaning the digestive tract at the same time. Pectin is one of the soluble fibres highly present in fruit.

Fibre should be obtained mainly from fruits and vegetables which should represent the bulk of a healthy diet, although an occasional treat of oatmeal or whole grain bread will also provide high percentages of fibre. Fibre-rich foods usually contain both types of fibre, but in different proportions specific to different foods.

Adding fibre to a diet that is made up mainly of refined foods in order to help increase the transit time in the digestive tract is not something that I would advise. Unhealthy foods (rice, bread, pasta, potatoes, pizzas, cakes, sweets, etc.) will still remain unhealthy even when fibre is added to the diet. This is why the only way to improve digestion, absorption and elimination is not to supplement your diet with extra fibre, but to eat natural foods full of protein, fibre, vitamins, minerals, enzymes, essential oils and water. Quick fix approaches never work in the long term; you have to be consistent in your nutritional approach and always eat the food that is ideal for human health. Too much extra or supplemented fibre can cause a lot of discomfort and loss of vitamins and minerals, which is followed by other negative health consequences. Although indigestible, fibre is still attacked by bacteria in the guts, causing methane gas to be released in a process that can cause bloating. Since fibre attracts a lot of water, it can pull water from the cells and disrupt the function of normal cells. This is why an increased consumption of fibre should always be accompanied by drinking enough water.

Our body benefits greatly from dietary fibre. If consumed through healthy natural food in daily amounts of 30 grams or more, dietary fibre will keep food moving faster through the digestive system, help our guts eliminate harmful bacteria quickly, keep the colon clean, prevent colon cancer, improve digestion and assimilation, maintain good health, lower the total blood cholesterol levels, and also help regulate normal blood sugar levels.

The bottom line

- Fibre is an essential component of natural food like fruits and veg-etables and has been a part of our diet throughout our evolution.
- Fibre is essential for maintaining good health; a lack of fibre can cause serious health problems.
- There are two types of dietary fibre: soluble and insoluble.
- They both help maintain the health of the colon and intestines.
- 30 grams of fibre in a daily diet is sufficient to promote good health.
- Diets consisting mainly of processed foods like bread, pasta, rice, potatoes, sweets, and cakes are poor in fibre and often cause con-stipation and other health problems.

Water

If we agree that oxygen is the most important element in supporting life, and that we cannot live without having access to oxygen (we can only stop breathing for a minute or so), we have to acknowledge that water is the next most important element that we have to consume in order to survive. Without food we can survive for 2 months or more, but without water we can't survive more than a few days!

Being the most important substance for survival after oxygen, water also comprises most of our body composition. Up to 75% of the human body is made of water. All of our tissues such as blood, muscles, skin; all our organs such as the heart, lungs, liver; all are made mostly of water. The water that we drink or that finds its way into the body through the food that we eat literally becomes us, a part of every single tissue and organ in our body.

Apart from composing our tissues and organs, water also plays a major role in the many different processes constantly happening in the body. Water helps digestion, absorption and elimination; regulates the body temperature when cooling and heating is distributed through perspiration and blood circulation; transports nutrients and oxygen to the cells; and helps the body to remove toxins and other by-products whilst being the biggest detoxifier. Water is involved in all chemical reactions in the body and, as such, is therefore involved in all metabolic processes. Water moves nutrients, hormones, antibodies and oxygen through the blood stream and also through the lymphatic system. Water even plays a role in joint lubrication.

In the absence of enough drinking water and natural food with a high water content (meats, fish, vegetables and fruits), and in the presence of some other liquids (alcohol, coffee, tea, fizzy drinks) or man-made processed foods (pasta, bread, pastries, pizzas, biscuits, sweets, cakes), dehydration occurs. Dehydration can cause many unwanted health consequences such as poor muscle tone, excess body fat, water retention, decreased digestive efficiency, decreased organ functions, stomach ulcers, toxin build-up, low energy, and more. Constipation is another common unwanted consequence of dehydration. Constipation can cause a build-up of toxins and lead to conditions like colon cancer, bowel cancer, lowered immunity, piles and other maladies.

One of the most common health problems today is water retention. An average person retains anywhere from 5-10 pounds (or more) of extra water. The causes may be different, such as eating too much salt or too many carbohydrates, taking different medications that cause water retention, high levels of stress, and more. But the most common cause of water retention is not drinking enough water and not eating enough natural food with a high water content.

If the body doesn't receive enough water on a daily basis, it will retain every drop of water that enters it in order to store it and protect itself, as the water deficiency is assumed part of the living environment. The best way to eliminate extra retained water that may cause numerous health problems, from high blood pressure to kidney problems, is to drink more water! Once the body starts receiving enough water, the reason for holding extra water will be eliminated and the body will be able to release it. Once it arrives in adequate quantities there is no reason to hold on it. Adequate water intake is important for everyone, but is especially important for people who exercise regularly. Perspiration and physical exercise increase the loss of water, which has to be replenished during and after exercise. It is also advisable to drink a glass (or two!) of water before you start exercising. During a training session (usually lasting from 45 to 60 minutes) up to one and a half litres of water should be drunk.

Exercising without drinking water can cause headaches, muscle fatigue, overall exhaustion and even muscle cramping. Drinking sugary drinks and so-called sport drinks while exercising is not my favourite option, however. These drinks are all saturated with sugar, sweeteners, colourings, acid and other elements that, altogether, require a lot of water in order to be dissolved and eliminated. Apart from that all these different components of sport drinks can cause water retention due to the body's hormonal response to them. Hormones like insulin will cause water retention themselves! So stick to drinking water during your training sessions, and eat properly in order to give the body all the necessary elements for muscular contractions. Your glycogen and mineral stores cannot be refilled with a single sports drink. It takes days before your training session for them to get full and ready for action.

Drinks such as coffee, tea, colas etc. have diuretic effects on the body, forcing the body to lose water and, even more importantly, minerals which are responsible for positive water balance in the body. Sodium and potassium — major players responsible for holding intra- and intercellular water in perfect balance — will always be lost due to the diuretic effects of the drinks mentioned above. If you are after an energetic, fully hydrated and healthy body, water should always be your preferred drink.

To be on the safe side, adults should drink at least 8 glasses of water per day. On hot summer days that amount should be increased. In addition, people who are physically active or who participate in sports should drink more than 8 glasses per day in order to satisfy the needs of the body, to hydrate properly, and to perform safely without suffering the consequences of dehydration. Increased perspiration, faster breathing, repetitive intense muscular contractions, and a faster metabolism while performing sports, all increase the demand for water well beyond the usual 8 glasses per day.

The bottom line

- Water is the major component of the human body. All body tissues are made up of water and water represents up to 75% of the human body.
- Water is necessary for all metabolic processes in the body.
- The human body cannot survive without water longer than a few days, while without food it can survive up to 2 months.
- We obtain necessary water from drinking water and from the food that we eat.
- Natural foods such as meat, fish, vegetables and fruits are rich in water and should make up the bulk of our diet. The content of water in these foods is as high as 90%.
- Grains are a very concentrated food and therefore have a very low percentage of water.
- All processed foods are concentrated and contain very little water.
- Dehydration can cause many unwanted health consequences such as stomach ulcers, toxin build-up, lowered immunity, etc.

Micronutrients

Micronutrients are elements which are essential to human nutrition but only required in minute amounts. Unlike macronutrients that are needed in hundreds of grams on a daily basis, micronutrients are only needed in amounts of around 20-100 milligrams or less per day. Although they have no caloric value (just like fats, proteins and carbohydrates), micronutrients are of essential importance when it comes to digesting and assimilating macronutrients. A deficiency in a single micronutrient will disrupt the optimal absorption of proteins, fats and/or carbohydrates. The complicated biochemical reactions involving hundreds of different chemicals to successfully complete digestion and absorption of nutrients require many different minerals, vitamins and trace elements. The overall efficiency of nutrient absorption greatly depends on the presence of all the essential micronutrients.

Vitamins, minerals and trace elements are all called micronutrients. They are all found in food and therefore their required amounts should be provided through balanced nutrition. Unfortunately, the large majority of the global population has no knowledge of or access to proper nutrition, and 2 billion people around the world (one third of the world's population) are estimated to suffer from micronutrient deficiency. Whilst the focus has been on providing enough food to the world's population, the quality and type of food that has been incorporated into staple diets has been compromised to a great extent. Malnutrition, for example, is not only caused by a lack of calories, but also by a lack of macronutrients in adequate balance and a lack of micronutrients in the correct amounts and necessary proportions that the body requires.

It is very well known that the lack of a single micronutrient can cause serious health problems in individuals, as well as in large sections of populations. A very common health problem caused by a deficiency of the micronutrient iron is anaemia. A deficiency in vitamin A causes xerophthalmia, while iodine deficiency causes goitre and cretinism. Other known conditions caused by a deficiency of a certain micronutrient are scurvy - caused by lack of vitamin C, pellagra - caused by deficiency of Niacin (vitamin B3), and beriberi - caused by lack of thiamine (vitamin B1).

Micronutrients work synergistically and must maintain a certain balance to provide optimum health. If some of them are not present in the amounts required to preserve the necessary balance in the body, health problems may occur. Whilst they are directly involved in enzyme production, a lack or inadequate amounts of one or a few of them can disrupt complicated enzyme production processes in the body and therefore affect the digestion of food and assimilation of nutrients, which will eventually lead to further health consequences.

Micronutrients are best consumed and assimilated in their perfect natural environment, which is natural fresh food. Fresh raw fruit and vegetables are the best source of vitamins, minerals and enzymes. Raw meat and fish also provide lots of vitamins, minerals and enzymes, but these substantially decrease during the processes of frying, roasting or boiling. Exposure to heat denaturalises enzymes, while thermo-unstable vitamins and some minerals lose their effectiveness once exposed to heat. Whilst fish (and especially meat, due to modern mass production) has to be cooked in order to be safe for human consumption, vegetables and fruit should be eaten in their natural state and raw. Only in this state they will provide us with all the necessary micronutrients needed for the perfect performance of all our body's systems.

If one is supplementing their diet with synthetic vitamins and minerals (not the best way to consume micronutrients), it is best to take them with food because components like macronutrients, enzymes, water and fibre increase the chances of micronutrient absorption. Micronutrients are there to aid the digestion and absorption of macronutrients in the first place. Their direct involvement in enzyme production and amino acid absorption, protection of essential oils from oxidation, carbohydrate absorption and other direct involvements in macronutrient absorption suggest strongly that supplements should not be taken without food (macronutrients) at the same time.

In recent times vitamins and minerals have been given mystical healing powers and often isolated from the whole process of body chemistry to which they are key contributors. Usually taken without food and in enormous amounts, vitamins and minerals can also be harmful to human health. As their name suggests, micronutrients work in very small amounts compared to macronutrients that are required in much larger quantities.

Processed foods, which have become the staple foods of modern societies, are very poor in the micronutrients essential to our health. Having been stripped of natural fibre, enzymes, vitamins and minerals through the processes of denaturing (cooking, drying, freezing, etc.), processed foods rob the body of essential micronutrients in order to be digested and absorbed, causing the body to become deficient in them. Unlike natural fresh foods that contain all the necessary micronutrients within them, processed foods such as all grains cereals, pastas, breads, rice, tinned foods, sweets, ready meals, etc., create an extra burden by creating micronutrient deficiencies. This is why food manufacturers often fortify these types of foods with extra vitamins and minerals in the hope that, through enrichment, they can bring the food closer to its natural state and make it more attractive to consumers. This approach can only be successful in food marketing; even with the extra-added micronutrients, the unhealthy and poor quality food will still be the same. Food is not meant to be "constructed" through the processes of denaturisation and then "fortified" after having been weakened; food is meant to be eaten in its full natural richness of macro and micronutrients.

Micronutrients still deliver the best results when ingested in the form of natural unprocessed foods. The absorption level of vitamins and minerals from fresh natural foods is optimal, whilst the absorption of synthetic vitamins and minerals from supplements is heavily compromised. For example, calcium found in dark green vegetables has the highest absorption rate, whilst calcium in supplements made from animal bones has a much lower absorption rate. This is the major reason for creating the "mega" supplements that contain extremely high dosages of vitamins and minerals, sometimes up to hundreds of times higher than our daily requirements. As we are not designed to eat bones, calcium from bones is absorbed at a much lower rate and therefore high dosage tablets are used to attempt to deliver the required amounts of daily calcium. Calcium from dark green fresh vegetables is absorbed at the highest levels, suggesting that a perfectly balanced diet with wholesome fresh foods contains the micronutrients necessary to satisfy our daily requirements. The problem that we are facing in our modern ultra-fast lives on this over-populated planet, where food has to be produced quickly and in huge amounts, is that we rarely eat perfect meals of the necessary quality on a regular basis. This is why supplements (meal replacements, protein shakes, protein bars, amino acids, and others) have found and secured their place in our modern diets.

Whilst in theory, eating wholesome "organically" grown food in the proper amounts and combinations will provide us with all the essential macro and micronutrients, in reality this rarely happens. Since so-called "organic" food has become another mass-produced food product and therefore has lost its "organic" nature, delivering higher amounts of vitamins and minerals than non-organic food has become questionable. We should therefore not have high expectations of these supermarket products. Organic food cannot be mass-produced, soils on which organic foods are grown cannot be forced to recover and deliver the same quality and amount of products season after season. The amounts of vitamins and minerals will never be the same in an apple grown in remote parts of the world where fertilisers and insecticides have never been used, and an apple grown in developed countries in soil that has been stripped of all its natural mineral resources and made dependent on synthetic fertilisers for decades.

Organic foods available in most markets today don't look different from non-organic foods, they don't taste different, and they have the same shape and same colours as non-organic foods. The only difference between organic and non-organic foods is in the labelling and in our belief that we are buying what is promised on the labels. Many of us remember how the apples looked from the trees in our grandmothers' gardens. It required a major effort to find two apples of the same size and colour; they smelled like apples from a distance and they tasted like no apple tastes today. They were definitely "organic", pecked by birds and attacked by insects; and those apples would have delivered many times more micronutrients than their heavily marketed and promoted hybrid organic cousins of today. The foods that most of us eat today either do not contain all of the necessary micronutrients or do not contain them in the proper amounts. This is one of the reasons why we have to supplement our food.

In my long fitness and life-coaching career, which has spanned more than twenty-five years, I have rarely seen people eating the right type of food in the right balance. Meals that are made mainly from fresh vegetables and lean protein sources, with the right amount of essential oils, are wishful thinking for thousands of people who have come to me seeking advice about nutrition, fitness, and life-style. Even the popular vegetarian way of eating is far from perfect, even further away than the common everyday eating approach. Ordinary people, even the ones who consider themselves health aware and health conscious, lack not only micronutrients, but also a massive amount of some essential macronutrients (water and fibre), and this has become far too commonplace in modern diets. Even people who have been actively engaged in recreational or professional sports are heavily lacking in many essential nutritional components such as protein, fibre, water, iron, vitamin C, vitamin B12, vitamin E and others.

Being honest and realistic, I would have to say that our diets today, as much as we think of them as perfect, require supplementation with extra minerals, vitamins, essential oils and sometimes with enzymes and proteins. It's not just because our food today is much poorer in micronutrients than the food that our ancestors used to eat, but that the pace of life, levels of stress, constant daily expectations to improve and deliver more, pollution and other modern life factors have put much higher demands on our bodies. In order to cope with these higher demands, our bodies are in constant need of micronutrients in the right balance and in the right levels. In our modern living environment, which is full of stress and pollution, we need them more than ever before. Although not the perfect solution, micronutrients in the form of supplements have become a reality. For this reason, enriching even the healthiest available food that we can get hold of today through supplements is a wise choice and a recommended practice.

The bottom line

- Vitamins, minerals and trace elements are called micronutrients.
- Micronutrients are essential elements in human nutrition.
- Micronutrients are directly involved in the absorption of macro-nutrients, and support the immune system and maintain the health of all the tissues in the body.
- Even the lack of a single micronutrient, over time, can cause serious health problems.
- Micronutrients work best in their natural environment, which is fresh food. Only in combination with other food components will they contribute with the highest efficiency to the body's metabolic processes.
- Food processing destroys most of the micronutrients present in fresh food.
- Micronutrients in the form of supplements are a necessity in our modern way of living. Taking into consideration the type of

food most of us eat nowadays and its quality and combination, environmental pollution, stress levels, and other factors, supplementing micronutrients that are well chosen and taken in the proper amounts on a daily basis will do us more good than harm.

Vitamins

Because they are micronutrients, vitamins are only needed in the body in minute amounts measured in milligrams or even micrograms. Even in such small amounts, however, vitamins are essential for sustaining life and maintaining health. Lack of just a single vitamin over a long period of time can cause serious health problems.

Vitamins have no caloric value and therefore the body cannot use them directly for energy or as building materials. Their essential role is in the production of enzymes, immune cells, blood, formation of skin and bone tissue and promotion of overall well-being. They are also called co-enzymes due to their direct involvement in enzyme production. Hundreds of enzymes and, consequently, the whole process of digestion and absorption depend on vitamins being present in the daily diet. These vitamins must also be consumed in the proper amount and proportion.

Vitamins can be split in two groups: water-soluble and fat-soluble. The majority of vitamins are water-soluble, meaning that they dissolve in water and are absorbed very quickly by the digestive system. Their constant presence in the body is only achieved through eating a few balanced meals during the day or by taking vitamin supplements. Any excess water-soluble vitamins will be eliminated through the urine, so there is no fear of the eventual toxicity of water-soluble vitamins, as they cannot be accumulated in the body.

Fat-soluble vitamins, on the other hand, can be accumulated in the body since they are stored in fat cells, and it is certainly a possibility that toxicity may result from taking too many supplements of these types of vitamins.

The daily requirements for vitamins have been established by the government and are known as the recommended daily allowance, or RDA. The problem with this though is that it is almost impossible to determine the right daily amount for every individual, simply because requirements change with gender, age, level of physical activity, stress levels, smoking, illness, infection and many other everyday life factors. The vitamin absorption threshold also changes in relation to the need for a certain vitamin. Individual requirements are very different and the only way to establish the correct amount is to experiment with regard to the above-mentioned factors. In comparison with the RDA of vitamins, actual daily requirements can sometimes be 20 times higher for certain vitamins in individuals who are over-stressed or involved in intense sport activities. In order to avoid over-taking supplements and experiencing unwanted side effects, a nutritionist's advice should be sought in determining your own specific vitamin requirements.

Although modern life forces us to require some supplements, fresh vegetables and fruits still have to compose the bulk of everyone's diet. Regardless of how much and how many different vitamins and minerals we can get through fresh foods, they are still most effective when their intake is through the consumption of healthy, natural food sources. Every single food item has different vitamins and miner-alsand different combinations in respect of relevant macronutrients, enzymes and other important components, and fish, meat and dairy products are also very rich sources of vitamins and minerals. As part of a balanced diet, protein sources have to secure their place in every meal of the day.

Now I would like to bring attention to the current addiction to pills and tablets. Living in a world run by media, and constantly surrounded by powerful marketing and advertising, we all long for a pill or tablet as a magic answer or solution for just about everything. We always want a magic pill that will keep our blood pressure or cholesterol down, or a contraceptive pill, a magic coenzyme, a most potent antioxidant, or a pill for cancer prevention; the list goes on and on. This is more than enough to create the pill-popping culture that we all see today. More and more people are getting heavily misled by the idea that pills can replace a healthy lifestyle, regular exercise, or well-balanced meals eaten at normal times in relaxed circumstances, not while driving or running to catch the bus.

I regularly meet clients who believe that, even if they don't eat well, they can still swallow a few handfuls of pills to compensate for abusing their bodies with junk food day after day. Supplements have to remain exactly what their name suggests: supplements! They must not - because they cannot - replace regular, well-balanced meals. The supplement industry constantly produces new products with such speed that I often meet clients who ask me about some new type of "pill" or supplement that I have never heard of before. The scenario I see is always the same: the average person suffers not from a lack of micronutrients in pill form, but a heavy lack of protein, essential fats, fibre and even water! Before you get into the right supplement program, make sure that you are eating the right type of food and that lean protein is a part of each daily meal. Make sure that the bulk of your diet consists of a variety of fresh vegetables, that you eat a few different fruits every day, and that you drink enough water. Supplements will only work if you are eating a proper diet in the first place, and remember that you should always take supplements together with your meals.

Vitamin A (Retinol)

Vitamin A belongs to the group of fat-soluble vitamins and therefore needs dietary fat in order to be properly metabolised. There are basically two forms in which vitamin A is found in nature. The type that can be directly used by the human body is called retinol and is found in animal sources such as fish oil and liver. In the case of plant sources, vitamin A can be manufactured by the body from substances contained in plants called carotenes. Good sources of carotenes include carrots and green leafy vegetables, while some other sources like yams and mangoes contain them in smaller amounts. Whilst the body can directly use retinol from animal sources, beta-carotenes cannot be used directly. They first have to be converted into retinol, but that is a very inefficient process because it takes up to 6 units of beta-carotenes to produce one unit of retinol.

Vitamin A can be stored in the liver and then used when needed, so toxicity of vitamin A is possible. However, deficiencies in vitamin A are common among people who eat very low-fat diets, or diets poor in vegetables. Since fat is needed for the absorption of vitamin A, low-fat diets can upset the delicate metabolism of it. Vitamin A deficiency is also common among vegetarians (which can cause problems with vision). Unfortunately, most vegetarians only think about avoiding animal protein sources, but in the process neglect the importance of a balanced diet (which for vegetarians is much more complicated) and miss out on a wide variety of other plant foods.

Vitamin A belongs to a group of chemicals known as antioxidants, whose main role is to fight free radicals, the most cell-damaging components in the body. Vitamin A is also involved in maintaining a healthy immune system and especially in protecting against infections of the eyes, ear, nose, throat, lungs and bladder. Vitamin A helps maintain good night vision, healthy skin and prevents acne and dermatitis.

The daily-recommended allowance of vitamin A is around 5 000 IU per day for adults. Higher dosages have been used without side effects (under 30 000 IU), but knowing that daily requirements vary among individuals depending on age, gender, health situations, physical activity and other factors, proper dosages can only be established through experimentation and consultation with a nutritionist.

Vitamin B Complex

B vitamins are found in nature in vegetables as well as in animal food. Some 16 different B vitamins have been isolated so far and they occur together in nature, which is why they are called B complex. They are water-soluble, which means that they dissolve in water and, because they act together in a certain balance, B vitamins have to be taken in the proper balance when supplemented. Overtaking a single B vitamin at the expense of others will disturb their delicate balance and their participation in major metabolic functions in the body.

The main role of B vitamins in the body is for the conversion of carbohydrates into glucose. They also strengthen the nervous system and help relieve symptoms of stress. B vitamins also help digestion, boost appetite, and fight anaemia, constipation and fatigue. The important thing to remember is to supplement them in proper balance with one another.

Vitamin B1 (Thiamin)

Being water-soluble, vitamin B1 cannot be stored in the body, so it has to be consumed daily through the diet or with supplements. Its major role in the body is to convert carbohydrates into glucose. The best natural sources of vitamin B1 are whole grains, rice bran, green vegetables and fruit. Sugar and white flour, alcohol and antibiotics can hinder the absorption of vitamin B1.

Thiamin is known to promote a feeling of well-being, overcome depression and emotional stress, improve appetite and aid digestion. A deficiency of vitamin B1 can cause neurosis, irritability, fear and anxiety. Low thyroid function and loss of appetite are also consequences of thiamin deficiency. Prolonged deficiency can cause beriberi.

Although the daily required amount is thought to be around 1.5 mg for adults, dosages of 50 mg daily have been proven to be much more effective. Toxicity of thiamin has not been reported for daily dosages under 500 mg.

Vitamin B2 (Riboflavin)

This is another B vitamin that has to be taken daily because of the body's inability to store water-soluble vitamins. The best sources of riboflavin are meats, poultry, fish and dairy products. It is involved in the break-down of carbohydrates, fats and proteins, helping the mitochondria of the muscles to burn energy. Riboflavin has also been found to help maintain good vision, healthy skin, hair and nails. It also promotes growth and fertility.

The daily recommended dosage is thought to be 1.7 mg but dosages of around 50 mg per day have been shown to be more beneficial.

Vitamin B3 (Niacin)

Niacin can be obtained through food or partly supplied by tryptophan in the diet which the body can convert into niacin. Some amounts of niacin can be stored in the liver, but they can get easily depleted when over-eating sugary food. Niacin is heat resistant so maintains its presence in food even after cooking. The best natural sources of vitamin B3 are meats and fish, liver, eggs and brewer's yeast. Niacin is also involved in the glycogen energy cycle, oxidation of fatty acids for energy and is also essential for the synthesis of sex hormones.

The daily requirements are around 19 mg, but dosages between 30 and 100 mg, especially in athletes, have been proven to be beneficial.

Vitamin B5 (Pantothenic Acid)

Pantothenic acid is found widely in most of the foods we eat on a daily basis; a deficiency of this vitamin is usually linked to serious calorie deprivation. Although not very common, a vitamin B5 deficiency can cause low blood-sugar levels, exhaustion and low adrenalin production. Pantothenic acid is necessary for the manufacture of glucose and fatty acids, which are the main fuels of the body. It also stimulates adrenal functions, prevents fatigue and reduces stress. The best natural sources of B5 are meat, liver, raw wheatgerm, beans and whole grains.

Estimated daily requirements are around 10 mg; supplemented dosages of around 50 mg have been shown to be more beneficial, especially in people involved in active sports.

Vitamin B6 (Pyroxidine)

Vitamin B6 takes part in many activities in the body. It helps release glycogen from the liver and the muscle tissues wherever energy is needed. Pyrodoxine also plays an essential role in the metabolism of essential fatty acids, and in regard to protein functions at all levels of protein and amino acid metabolism. It also helps in the manufacture of haemoglobin. Because vitamin B6 cannot be stored in the body, deficiency is common, especially among dieters and people who often fast. Some of the symptoms of deficiency are hypoglycaemia, appetite loss, high cholesterol levels, allergies, and water retention.

The best natural sources are liver, kidney, eggs and brewer's yeast. The daily recommended dosage is estimated to be 2.2 mg, but it can be supplemented safely up to 100 mg per day.

Vitamin B12 (Cyanocobalamin)

Although the minuscule requirements for vitamin B12 are measured in mcg (micrograms) whilst other B vitamins are measured in mg (milligrams), vitamin B12 represents the most important vitamin in the B group. It occurs in meat, liver and eggs, and cannot be found in plants. This is why strict vegetarians generally suffer from B12 deficiency. Vegetarians who include eggs and dairy products in their daily diet are much better off with regards to the necessary consumption of this essential micronutrient. Vitamin B12 forms part of the coenzymes essential for all cells, particularly red blood cells, cells of the lining of the gastrointestinal tract and bone marrow cells. It contributes to the formation of red blood cells in the bone marrow and therefore prevents anaemia, increases energy levels, helps maintain a healthy nervous system and also promotes growth and appetite in children. It also helps the action of other vitamins from the B group and also vitamin C.

The daily recommended dosage is around 3 mcg. Through supplements you can safely take up to 100 mcg in order to ensure maximum benefit of this very important vitamin.

Folate (Folic Acid)

This is another vitamin from the B group that is measured in mcg (micrograms). This vitamin is easily destroyed by heat - so cooked vegetables are simply stripped of this essential vitamin. Together with vitamin B12, folic acid takes part in the synthesis of nucleic acids and also in the metabolism of amino acids.

A deficiency in folic acid inhibits the growth of new cells and can also cause a loss of appetite, depression and digestive problems. The best sources of folic acid are dark green and leafy vegetables, liver, beans and carrots. The daily requirements are thought to be around 400 mcg.

Biotin

Biotin is essential for the formation of new glucose and fatty acid synthesis, which are two major fuels for energy. A deficiency in biotin leaves a person without the ability to build new proteins and this can manifest in the loss of hair and muscle tissue, adverse skin conditions, a lack of appetite and fatigue.

Avidin, a component found in raw eggs, or more precisely in raw egg whites, disrupts the body's absorption of biotin and causes its deficiency. This is the main reason why eggs should be eaten cooked and not raw. The best natural sources of biotin are liver, egg yolks, brown rice and fruit. The daily recommended dosage of biotin is around 300 mcg.

Choline

Although the body can make choline from the amino acid methionin, the primary source of choline is still food. It forms part of lecithin, an important component of the membrane of every single cell in the body. Choline is lipotropic, which means that it is involved in the emulsification of fat and also in the utilisation of fat and cholesterol. Choline can also lower cholesterol, improve memory and learning ability, and keeps the liver healthy. A deficiency of choline can cause fatty degeneration of the liver and high cholesterol. Choline is found in eggs, liver, brains and green leafy vegetables.

The average recommended daily amount of choline from food is thought to be around 900 mg.

Inositol

Inositol, like choline, is also involved in the formation of lecithin and thus is lipotropic and involved in the metabolism of fat and cholesterol. Inositol plays an important role in the normal metabolism of calcium and insulin, and can also lower cholesterol in the liver. It is believed that inositol has a calming effect and can improve one's overall mental state. A deficiency of inositol can cause hypertension, high cholesterol levels, and skin problems.

Inositol is found in liver and brewer's yeast. Although the daily required amount has still not been established, nutritionists recommend daily supplements in the amount of 1 g.

Vitamin C (Ascorbic Acid)

Vitamin C deserves to be called a super-vitamin, simply because of its vast and significant role in the body. Not only does vitamin C play an essential role in the metabolism of amino acids, but in strengthening immunity too, detoxifying the body, combating tissue aging and supporting health overall.

Vitamin C is a water-soluble vitamin and is very unstable. The human body cannot synthesise and store it, so it has to be taken daily. However, because vitamin C leaves the body within 4 hours after consumption, it should be ingested through food or supplements every 4 hours. Cooking, boiling, and peeling the skin off fruits will all destroy vitamin C.

Vitamin C is one of the most potent detoxifiers. It helps the body to get rid of toxic elements like lead, copper and mercury. It also helps eliminate many different carcinogens that enter the body via food, alcohol or smoking. One of its most important roles in the body is to form collagen, which is the main component of all connective tissues in the body. Strong connective tissues are of utmost importance for physical performance, stability and longevity. Reduced collagen will interfere with the strength of connective tissues, causing many unwanted health problems. Wrinkling of the skin is just one example of reduced collagen production.

Vitamin C aids the absorption of calcium and iron in the body as well as of certain amino acids. It also provides an immunity boost and is important for boosting leukocyte functions for fighting infections. It prevents viruses from entering the body by helping with the production of interferon. It has also been found to be very helpful in impairing the growth of some tumours and lowering the risk of some types of cancer like cancer of the mouth, lung, stomach, colon and breast. Mega-doses of vitamin C can also prolong the life of cancer patients. Vitamin C suppresses the high production of cortisol, supporting a stronger testosterone to cortisol ratio that is especially important for people who are active in sports. It helps the healing of wounds, strengthens the capillaries and blood vessels, promotes healthy gums and teeth and relieves depression. Finally, vitamin C has been found to lower cholesterol levels in the body, and it strengthens the arteries reducing the risk of arteriosclerosis.

Deficiency of vitamin C increases the chances of infections and allergies, and causes scurvy, bleeding of the gums, depression, anxiety, wrinkling of the skin, loss of appetite, and anaemia. The best natural sources are dark green vegetables, tomatoes, strawberries, and citrus fruits. Vitamin C functions best in the presence of bioflavonoids, substances that occur naturally in foods rich in vitamin C so if taken as a supplement, take it along with bioflavonoids.

The recommended daily dosages are estimated to be around 60 mg, but supplements of 3-4 grams per day have been proven to be more beneficial in order to prevent infections and support an active lifestyle. During colds, infections, high stress, intense sports and low calorie dieting, the daily dosage of vitamin C may go as high as 8 grams per day. High amounts of daily vitamin C intake should be supported by extra intake of magnesium.

Vitamin D

Vitamin D is a fat-soluble vitamin and its daily needs in the body are measured in mcg (micrograms) or IU (international units). There are two ways of getting the necessary amounts of vitamin D: one is through food and the other is from sunlight. Under direct exposure to sunlight our skin can manufacture vitamin D. By using cholesterol under the skin, the body can synthesise vitamin D, which is then directly absorbed into the bloodstream. Upon absorption vitamin D is stored in the liver and then delivered wherever it is required. People who don't get direct exposure to sunlight have to consider a better diet or adequate supplements of vitamin D.

The major role of vitamin D is to regulate calcium absorption. It's responsible for getting calcium into the bloodstream and delivering it to the bones. A deficiency of vitamin D can cause soft and brittle bones and also weak teeth. A long-term deficiency in children can also cause rickets.

The best natural sources are fish liver oil, salmon, tuna, sardines and herring. The required daily amount is thought to be around 400 IU.

Vitamin E

Vitamin E is a fat-soluble vitamin measured in IU (international units). It comes in many forms; alpha tocopherol is the most potent antioxidant in the human body and, as such, plays a major role in protecting all cell membranes in the body from damaging oxidative processes, especially of polyunsaturated essential fatty acids. An increased intake of essential fatty acids in the form of omega-3 would require an adequate increase in vitamin E intake to prevent them from oxidizing and forming damaging free radicals. Free radicals are known to weaken immunity and also damage the DNA of cells, potentially leading to cancer. Lymphocytes and neutrophils, the most common type of white blood cells, contain 10-20 times more vitamin E than red blood cells, suggesting the importance of vitamin E for their activities. Neutrophils represent 50-70 % of white blood cells and are the first immune cells called on to fight infection. Vitamin E can also help protect against blood clotting and therefore protect against arteriosclerosis and heart attack. Vitamin E can also help prevent coronary heart disease by limiting oxidation of LDL-cholesterol.

Research has shown that people who regularly take vitamin E lower their risk of getting cardiovascular diseases by up to 40% compared to people who don't take vitamin E. Vitamin E improves blood circulation and has the ability to thin the blood, and also prevents the formation of blood clots. Being one of the most potent antioxidants, vitamin E helps cell regeneration and slows ageing of all tissues in the body. It also increases fertility and helps maintain a healthy sexual drive. Vitamin E protects against pollutants that enter the body through food, water and air, being a strong detoxifier.

The best natural sources of vitamin E are vegetable oils, whole grains, nuts, green leafy vegetables and eggs. The daily requirements are 15 IU, while supplements of up to 800 IU have been shown to be very beneficial. People who are actively involved in sports and intense physical activity need more vitamin E in order to fight the increased production of free radicals.

Vitamin K

Vitamin K is a fat-soluble vitamin that plays a crucial role in the coagulation of blood. Without the action of vitamin K, blood would not clot and even small wounds would cause unstoppable bleeding. Vitamin K also helps in preventing soft tissue calcification, especially cartilage, and also strengthens bone tissue.

The best natural sources of vitamin K are green leafy vegetables. The daily requirements are between 150 and 300 mcg, which are usually supplied by daily food intake.

Vitamin P

Vitamin P is actually another name for the group of substances known as bioflavonoids. Bioflavonoids are water-soluble and, in plants, are always present along with vitamin C. Bioflavonoids enhance the action and absorption of ascorbic acid and there are hun-

dreds of different kinds - rutin and quercetin being two of the most potent. Rutin aids the absorption of vitamin C, preserving the structure of capillaries and preventing bleeding and bruising. It also has an antibacterial effect and promotes circulation. Quercetin has been found to be one of the most active bioflavonoids and a very strong antioxidant and antihistamine having a very strong anti-inflammatory effect. Quercetin has also been found to be a potent anti-viral chemical and may also prevent cancer, especially prostate cancer.
The best natural sources are citrus fruits. Ideally bioflavonoids should be present in an amount equal to one-fifth of the amount of vitamin C.

Coenzyme Q10

Coenzyme Q10 is a fat-soluble, vitamin-like substance that is found in every human cell. It is essential because of its involvement in mitochondria for most of the energy production in the human body.

Coenzyme Q10 is a powerful antioxidant and prevents oxidation of the fatty acids protecting the cell membranes. Coenzyme Q10 is found in high concentration in the human heart, suggesting the high importance of this substance in regulating a healthy heart. Research has shown that Q10 has a beneficial effect in strengthening the heart muscle and lowering high blood pressure. Other benefits of Q10 are the promotion of gum health, enhanced activity of the white blood cells, improved immunity and longevity. The best natural sources of coenzyme Q10 are organ meats: heart, liver, kidney, beef; sardines and mackerel; and polyunsaturated vegetable oils.

The Bottom Line

- Vitamins are essential food components needed in very small amounts on a daily basis. They are measured in micrograms and milligrams.
- Lack of a single vitamin can lead to serious health consequences.
- Vitamins are found in fresh vegetables, fruit, fish and meat.
- Food processing destroys most of the vitamins found in fresh food.
- Vitamins can be split in two groups: water-soluble and fat-soluble.
- Whilst water-soluble vitamins are excreted daily if taken in higher than needed amounts, fat-soluble vitamins can accumulate in different tissues in the body and cause toxic reactions if taken in higher amounts than needed.
- The daily requirements for vitamins vary depending on many factors such as age, physical activity, lean body weight, stress levels, etc.
- Vitamins in the form of supplements should not be overly relied upon compared to vitamins found in fresh food. Fresh food should comprise the bulk of our diet, while supplements can only come second.

Macrominerals

Minerals are the substances that enable all metabolic processes in the body, and they must to be supplied to us on a continual daily basis in order to allow healthy metabolic functions. Minerals work in synergy; if even one of them is lacking in the diet, the complex mineral participation in all chemical processes in the body can be disturbed and cause health problems.

Although minerals should be present naturally in most of the foods that we eat on a daily basis, there are many different factors determining which minerals will be present and in what amounts. Minerals which are supposed to be present in some fruits and vegetables are not always present in the exact numbers and amounts expected. Intense farming over many decades depletes the soil of many minerals, which is later reflected in foods that are lacking in essential minerals. In many remote regions of the world where soils are not depleted and plants have not been sprayed with chemicals such as pesticides or herbicides, people live long lives and benefit from good health; the food that they eat regularly is full of the essential minerals that help them develop strong immune systems and live longer lives. Soil depletion is one of the major reasons why the everyday diet in developed countries has to be supplemented with extra minerals and vitamins. There are also other life factors that can disrupt mineral absorption and cause mineral deficiency; poor diet, stress, illness, infection, injuries, alcohol and smoking are all factors that create adverse hormonal reactions and also require greater amounts of minerals and vitamins in order to restore normal physical health and synergy.

Essentially, there are 2 major types of minerals: macrominerals and trace elements. Macrominerals are: calcium, phosphorus, potassium, magnesium, sodium and sulphur. Trace elements are: iron, zinc, copper, manganese, chromium, selenium, iodine, fluorine, molybdenum, silica, boron and germanium.

Macrominerals are present in the body in amounts over 5 grams and our daily intake requirements are over 100 mg. Trace elements are minerals that are found in the body in much smaller quantities, and our daily requirements are under 100 mg. Although found in the body and needed in much smaller amounts than macrominerals, trace elements are no less important to us. A deficiency in a single trace element can cause major health problems by disrupting enzyme production and/or mineral and vitamin absorption. This is why macrominerals and trace elements have to be taken in the right amounts and in perfect balance. Supplementing just one macromineral or trace element in mega amounts (a common practice among the misinformed) does not result in a positive effect.

Calcium

Calcium is by far the most abundant mineral in the body. The average person's body weighing 80 kg contains about 1.5 kg of calcium. 99% of that amount is stored in the bones and teeth. The remaining 1% plays a crucial role in the body by controlling nerve impulses, contraction of the skeletal muscles, heartbeat, blood clotting and more. The importance of constantly maintaining that 1% within very tight limits is overwhelming, so when the intake of calcium in the daily diet is not sufficient, the body has to raid bone tissue and pull calcium out of the bones in order to satisfy more essential life functions.

Optimal calcium absorption doesn't only depend on regular and adequate calcium intake, but also on proper daily supplies of vitamin D, phosphorus, magnesium, zinc, vitamin A, vitamin C and adequate production of stomach acid. Once again, the synergy of all these essential vitamins and minerals is of great importance.

In cases of calcium deficiency or low absorption capability, the result is porous and brittle bones. This condition is especially common in women, who frequently suffer from osteoporosis. What has often been overlooked when discussing the absorption of calcium and the strengthening of bones is the fact that bones have to be continually stressed in order to preserve more calcium and stay strong. Unless they are continually stressed, their structure weakens, which is where strength training steps in. Weight training is the best way of strengthening and increasing muscle tissue, which in turn directly strengthens the bones. The more muscle tissue present, the stronger the bones, and the less muscle tissue, the weaker the bones, which is what usually happens as we grow older.

Whilst strength training offers the best possible way to strengthen the bones, athletes have often shown a deficiency in calcium because bone mineralization increases greatly in response to the stress of exercise. In the case of active sports, especially in strength training, the daily intake of calcium and other relevant microelements has to increase. Athletes have higher requirements for essential minerals and vitamins than non-athletes. Higher protein consumption, common in strength sports, also causes increased calcium exertion and requires additional calcium supplements supported with other micronutrients. A serious consequence of calcium deficiency is high blood pressure; other symptoms include, amongst other things, tooth decay, muscle cramps and aches, and skin disorders.

The best natural sources of calcium are dairy products and dark green vegetables. People allergic to lactose should consider calcium supplements. The daily requirement for calcium is 1 000 mg, but that increases with heavy sports activity, lactation, pregnancy and old age.

Phosphorus

There are around 800 grams of phosphorus in the average-sized adult body. Most of it, around 700 grams, is contained in the bones, whilst the rest is used by the body for essential enzymatic and chemical processes. Phosphorus is involved in energy formation in the body in the form of glycogen, which is the energy stored in the liver and muscles. Phosphorus maintains strong bones and teeth and promotes growth and tissue repair.

The nucleic acids DNA and RNA, which are responsible for the storage and transmission of genetic information, are long chains of phosphate-containing molecules. Phosphorus is also involved in the activation of many enzymes and hormones. Phosphorus helps to maintain a normal acid-base balance (pH) by acting as one of the body's most important acid buffers. It is also involved in building haemoglobin in red blood cells, and affects oxygen delivery to all the tissues in the body.

The proper balance between phosphorus and calcium is a ratio of 1 to 2.5. This balance helps ensure optimum mineralization of the bones. The best natural food sources of phosphorus are meat, fish, eggs and whole grains. The daily recommended intake is around 1 000 mg and this amount is usually obtainable through a balanced diet.

Magnesium

Most of the body's magnesium is contained in the skeleton (around 60%) while the remaining amount is contained in the soft tissues. Magnesium forms part of over 300 enzymes in the body and is involved in ATP (adenosine triphosphate) production for energy in the muscles. This important mineral also regulates muscle contractions including the heartbeat. Magnesium hardens the enamel that protects the teeth from decay. It is found in the bones in a 1 to 2 proportion to calcium. The increased need for calcium in athletes requires an increased consumption of magnesium in order to keep the preferred balance of 1 to 2.

Magnesium is excreted in sweat, so people who perspire heavily, such as athletes, need to consider consuming the right amount of magnesium in order to replenish their magnesium stores. Athletes are often deficient in magnesium.

Magnesium prevents build-up of kidney stones by keeping the calcium soluble, so an increased intake of calcium should be accompanied by an increased intake of magnesium, to ensure that the two minerals always remain in the right balance.

The best food sources of magnesium are legumes and whole grains. The daily recommended amount is round 350 mg, whilst people who are actively engaged in sports will benefit from supplementing their diet and taking up to 1 000 mg of magnesium daily. Alcohol consumption depletes magnesium from the body, so if you drink regularly (which is obviously not advisable), consider supplementing your diet with this important mineral.

Sodium

The three main electrolytes in the body are sodium, potassium and chloride. They perform essential electrochemical reactions in the body, without which human life wouldn't be possible. In order to perform perfectly, electrolytes have to be present in the body in a perfect balance. Under-supply of one or over-consumption of another can cause electrolyte imbalance with negative health consequences.

Sodium is the main positively-charged electrolyte outside the cells. It is the primary regulator of the fluid in extra-cellular space, which is the space between the cells. The balance of fluid in the body greatly depends on sodium. It helps regulate pH balance and helps active transport of nutrients to all cells of the body. Sodium is also a crucial substance in regulating osmotic pressure in the body, which controls the essential supply and excretion of nutrients through the cell membranes of every cell in the body.

Sodium tends to cause water retention in the body and increases blood pressure when taken in high amounts. Although sodium deficiency is rare, it can cause weight loss, fatigue and dehydration. Sodium is present in all the foods that we eat, so adding it to food in the form of table salt is really not necessary. The best natural sources of sodium are fish, meats, eggs, apples, carrots, and cabbage. The recommended daily amount is up to 3 grams.

Potassium

Whilst sodium controls the fluids outside the cells, potassium, as the main positively-charged electrolyte inside the cells, takes control of the intracellular fluids. Together with sodium, potassium creates a so-called "sodium-potassium pump" that moves the fluids containing nutrients back and forth between the interior and exterior of the cell. This essential role of the pump regulates the correct sodium-potassium balance and stimulates kidney function, maintaining nerve functions and muscle contractions.

In our modern diets, overwhelmed by processed foods which are very high in sodium, the balance between potassium and sodium is 1 to 3. In most natural foods the balance between potassium and sodium is about 7 to 1. In order to preserve the healthy balance of potassium and sodium, we should eat mainly natural fresh food and avoid processed foods, which are usually over-salted.

The best natural sources of potassium are meats, fish, almonds, apples, and green leafy vegetables, although it is present in most fruit and vegetables. The recommended daily requirements are about 3.5 grams, although potassium is not toxic up to 5 grams a day. People involved in sports may benefit from potassium supplements, as perspiration depletes potassium.

Trace Elements

Iron

The major role of iron is to form part of the haemoglobin, the red pigment which carries oxygen in the blood from the lungs to the muscles, brain and other body tissues. Without iron, brain cells would simply die from a lack of oxygen. Haemoglobin is also responsible for transporting carbon dioxide from the tissues to the lungs where it is exhaled. Iron is also involved in the production of many essential enzymes. The amount of the iron stored in the body is around 5 grams.

Deficiencies of iron are quite common thanks to the body's low absorption of this essential trace mineral. Although iron is found in whole grains, vegetables, and eggs, heme iron from meat is the most bio-available and absorbable. However, even the best heme iron from meat is only absorbable at a rate of 10%! Iron found in vegetables is only 1% bio-available! In order to increase the absorption of iron it is important to supplement the diet with other micronutrients like vitamins C and B12.

A deficiency of iron can cause anaemia, which is a decrease in red blood cells or haemoglobin levels, impairing the ability of the blood to transport oxygen. Women lose more iron than men due to the monthly menstrual cycle and pregnancy, and therefore require a higher daily iron intake than men. People regularly engaged in intense sport activities also need more iron on a daily basis.

The best natural sources of iron are liver, meats, eggs, whole grains and green leafy vegetables. The recommended daily intake for iron is 10 mg for men and 18 mg for women.

Zinc

Zinc is a component of over 25 different enzymes, and thousands of different functions in the body involve zinc. However, only 1.8 grams is stored in the body and it can easily be depleted so has to be supplied daily, either from food or via supplements.

Zinc is also involved in the action of several hormones such as testosterone, oestrogen, insulin and growth hormone. It plays an essential role in the functions of the reproductive system, and especially in maintaining the health and proper functioning of the prostate gland in men. Adequate and regular zinc supplies are essential for normal testosterone levels and sperm counts. Incidences of impotence are partially caused by chronic zinc deficiency.

Athletes need to pay special attention to regular zinc intake because of the higher production of red blood cells, loss of zinc through perspiration, increased fatty acid metabolism and higher testosterone needs associated with increased physical activity.

Although severe zinc deficiencies are not very common, the majority of people's daily zinc intake is below daily requirements. Smoking and drinking are known to deplete the body's zinc reserves. The best natural sources of zinc are meat, fish, oysters, walnuts, eggs and green leafy vegetables. The daily requirement for zinc is 15 mg, but athletes should supplement zinc up to 50 mg per day.

Copper

Copper is a trace element that is needed in the body in very small amounts. Nonetheless, copper plays an important role in the function of many enzymes, being involved in the production of nor-adrenalin, an enzyme that controls cross-linking of collagen and elastin, the connective tissues in the body. Copper is also involved in functions of the enzyme "superoxide dismutase" (SOD), one of the most powerful free-radical eliminators in the body. It also aids the absorption of iron, and therefore supports production of haemoglobin.

An accumulation of excess copper in the body can cause many unwanted side effects such as hypertension, depression and arthritis, amongst others. Copper deficiency can cause anaemia, weakening of the aorta and fatigue.

The best natural sources are organ meats and seafood. The recommended daily requirement for copper is 3 mg.

Manganese

Manganese helps maintain healthy bones and cartilage. It is also involved in the activation of many of the enzymes that regulate carbohydrate metabolism and blood sugar levels. It helps production of thyroxin, the major thyroid hormone, and increases activity of one of the most potent anti-oxidants, superoxide dismutase (SOD). Manganese also takes part in the synthesis of cholesterol and fatty acids.

The best natural sources of manganese are nuts, whole grains and green leafy vegetables. The recommended daily intake of manganese is between 2 and 5 mg. In cases of muscle injury or inflammation, supplements of up to 100 mg per day for 2 weeks can be beneficial.

Chromium

Chromium is one of the essential trace elements that play a key role in the body's ability to enhance insulin functions, especially those related to glucose levels in the blood. Being essential for the normal metabolism of glucose, insulin, cholesterol and fatty acids, as well as muscle growth, a chromium-rich diet has to be considered by diabetics and people with cholesterol and glucose tolerance problems.

Modern diets, high in sugar and products made of white flour, are the major cause of chromium deficiency which is widespread among people whose major food choice is refined carbohydrates. Sugar, providing only empty calories by itself, needs many different vitamins, minerals, and trace elements in order to be digested and absorbed. Chromium is one of these essential micronutrients that gets depleted by high sugar intake. Years of poor lifestyle practices and improper diet can bring the body to a situation where chromium deficiency creates conditions like glucose intolerance, hypoglycaemia, insulin resistance and eventually diabetes.

The best form of supplemental chromium is chromium picolinate, which has the highest absorption level and is shown to lower glucose and cholesterol levels in the body. Not only can chromium picolinate help in losing fat, but it also helps by increasing muscle tissue in athletes. The best natural sources are brewer's yeast, meat and shellfish. It is estimated that the optimal dosage for the general population is 200 mcg, while athletes can supplement up to 500 mcg of chromium.

Selenium

Selenium is one of the body's most potent anti-oxidants. It is also an integral component of the very powerful anti-aging and antioxidant enzyme called glutathione peroxidase, which destroys damaging free radicals called hydroperoxidase. Selenium is found to provide many health benefits such as decreased rates of cancer and heart attack and improved immunity. Most of these properties are due to selenium's high antioxidant potency.

Selenium works best in the presence of vitamin E, another very strong antioxidant. Selenium deficiency can cause premature ageing, potential risk of cancer and heart attack.

The best natural sources of selenium are tuna, brewer's yeast, nuts and seeds. The daily recommended amount from food or supplements is around 200 mcg.

Iodine

Iodine is a trace element critical for the production of thyroid hormones, which control all energy in the body, metabolic rate, prevent accumulation of cholesterol and burn excess body fat. In the case of iodine deficiency, the thyroid gland grows new cells in order to produce more thyroxin and increases in size, causing the condition known as goitre. Iodine deficiency also causes mental retardation, cretinism, growth retardation and intellectual disability.

Although only necessary in small amounts in the body (around 25 mg), iodine plays an essential role in the overall health of an individual. Deficiency is rare these days thanks to iodised salt (a process started in 1920), but excessive perspiration can disturb the delicate amount of iodine in the body.

The best natural source is any type of seafood and of course, iodised salt. The RDA (recommended daily amount) of iodine is about 150 mcg daily.

Other Trace Elements

In addition to the above-mentioned trace elements, there are also others that contribute to overall health and well-being.

Fluorine is another non-metallic essential trace element that is necessary for the formation of strong teeth and bones. Fluorine increases resistance to tooth decay and bone fractures. The best sources of fluorine are seafood and fluoridated water.

Cobalt is another important trace element that represents an essential part of vitamin B12.

Boron, a non-metallic trace element promotes absorption of calcium and magnesium, prevents osteoporosis and helps growth.

Molybdenum is an essential part in the formation of many enzymes involved in different processes in the body.

Germanium is another potent antioxidant that protects the body from some types of cancers, leukaemia, diabetes, digestive problems and hypertension.

The bottom line

- Minerals are essential micro components found in food.
- They are found in natural fresh food; food processing depletes the minerals found in fresh food.
- Minerals are involved in many vital processes in the body from enzyme formation, bone strength, and water content in the tissues to oxygen transfer and many other processes.
- Mineral deficiencies cause serious health problems.
- Factors such as illnesses, injuries, alcohol, smoking, improper diet, stress etc. can cause mineral deficiency.
- Minerals can be categorized either as bulk minerals or trace elements.

Enzymes

What are enzymes?

Enzymes are protein-based chemicals which control metabolic processes in the body. They act as catalysts by starting or speeding up chemical reactions without undergoing any change themselves. Enzymes are present in every single cell of the body and in every living cell in the animal and plant world. Life simply wouldn't be possible without enzymes and their powerful role in the processes of life. Natural food is full of enzymes. Fruit, vegetables, fish and meat in their fresh, natural state are buzzing with them. Eaten in their fresh state, these foods provide the body with an abundance of different enzymes which help the body strengthen immunity and prolong life. They are involved in the digestion of food, the strengthening of the immune system, in controlling energy processes in the body, repairing tissues and many more essential metabolic functions. Supplied through healthy and fresh food, enzymes preserve the body's own enzyme production, allowing the huge amount of body energy that would otherwise be needed for this to be used instead to facilitate immune functions and many other bodily processes.

When food is depleted of enzymes, the body has to produce a large amount of them in order to digest and metabolise the very same food. Because of this, the body can be put under massive pressure to produce the right enzymes in adequate amounts, which requires a great deal of extra energy. Spending most of its life energy to produce enzymes and digest unhealthy "dead" food, the body has less energy available to protect itself and immunity weakens. No wonder that people who mainly eat food that is empty in enzymes, such as fast foods and processed foods, often get infections, feel sick, experience constant weakness and also suffer from illnesses of various organs.

Enzymes control all anabolic and catabolic processes in the body; anabolism refers to the process of building more complex substances from simpler ones and catabolism means breaking down complex substances into simpler parts. These processes together form our overall metabolism, which is controlled by thousands of different enzymes without which life would not be possible.

In our pill and fast food culture, where we expect almost everything to be given to us hassle-free at any time we want, we often forget that a pill cannot cure every health problem and nothing healthy can be delivered in a packed, pre-cooked lunch. Although they may be convenient, quick to prepare and can even taste great, precooked foods, dried foods, frozen foods and other similar processed foods will never deliver all the goodness found in natural, fresh, unprocessed produce.

Whatever supplements we take in the form of a pill will always be micronutrients —such as vitamins, minerals and trace elements. These "extras" can only supplement something that is much more important for our survival and healthy living, macronutrients. Without macronutrients (proteins, fats and carbohydrates) micronutrients would have no value because they would have nothing to interact with. However, apart from containing essential macronutrients, natural foods also contain something else that is of great importance for our health and well-being. These are enzymes, which help us digest food better, fight diseases, have more energy and live longer.

Did you ever suffer from indigestion, a gas build-up that makes you feel uncomfortable, or maybe from heartburn, allergies, lethargy, skin problems, weight problems or other similar maladies? If the answer is yes (which is most likely the answer for the majority of people), what was your first reaction to these problems? I'm quite positive that most people would expect that some medicine in the form of a pill would be the answer, that it would make you feel better and help you carry on with your daily routine. But how long would it really help for? There is another way of dealing with these kinds of problems. The first thing to do is to assess your lifestyle and the food that you are eating during the course of each day.

The most common food eaten by the majority of people is made of highly refined foods — edibles that supply only empty calories, with lots of salt, sugar or oil. These, as well as flavourings and other ingredients, are added to the basic refined components in order to make them tasty and tempting to eat. They have nothing to do with natural food, which is the only food that we should eat as it has been created by nature for us. These cheap, flavoured edibles have been stripped of active ingredients that were present in their natural shape: mainly enzymes.

Enzyme-free food is what I like to call dead food; food that doesn't provide life-giving qualities; therefore food that doesn't support and prolong our own lives. The most common processed edibles which create havoc for our health are unfortunately part of the everyday eating habits of the majority of people - pastas, rice, bread, pastries, potatoes, sweets, cakes and every other edible containing white flour, processed starch, sugar and salt. The ingredients in these edibles have been processed so many times that they have been robbed of the many minerals, vitamins, fibre, and enzymes that they originally had in their natural state. On top of that, they have been dried, frozen, baked, cooked and exposed to very high or very low temperatures so that they have been totally denatured. Everything that has been provided in these foods by Mother Nature was taken away to create the commercially desirable long shelf life: food that can be stored for a long time, and transported from one corner of the world to another whilst, at the same time, preserving their caloric value and taste. Profit-wise they are perfect products, yet health-wise they are disasters. Natural foods have a very short life span and therefore a very short shelf life. They cannot be stored for long periods of time, or packed and squeezed in order to save space. They also require more time to eat.

Natural foods contain many different enzymes which not only cause them to ripen, but also cause them to rot. These enzymes, in a way, digest the foods until they disintegrate. The enzymes in natural foods are the biggest problem for food manufacturers and retailers, who have had to turn to science in order to eliminate them from foods in order to make these foods more profitable by extending their shelf life. Food devoid of enzymes is dead food and doesn't support or prolong life, or strengthen immunity. So why do the majority of people still eat this kind of food? The reasons are many, but the most important are that these kinds of foods are cheap, and that the public is not given the right information to make informed choices.

For centuries, people have known that eating fresh fruit and vegetables provides good health. The abundance of enzymes, co-enzymes and co-factors available in fresh fruit and vegetables is the key to preserving people's health and strengthening their immunity. Although nowadays we all know that eating 4 - 5 daily servings of fresh fruit and vegetables can dramatically decrease the chances of developing cardiovascular diseases, diabetes and cancer, still only about 10% of people eat 2 portions of fresh fruit or 3 portions of fresh vegetables per day! Around 50% of people do not eat fresh fruit and vegetables at all! These statistics are a perfect breeding ground for a health disaster!

There are many different types of enzymes that are involved in the processes of breathing, fighting free radicals, cell repair, thinking, digestion, etc. Digestive enzymes that are secreted once food enters the digestive system are the next subject of our attention in this book.

Digestive enzymes

Digestive enzymes are mainly catabolic enzymes because they help to break down food after it has been eaten. Once food is broken down into smaller pieces through chewing, the appropriate enzymes start their work, even in the mouth.

In order to properly digest and absorb the food that we eat, our bodies produce different enzymes that target different macronutrients such as protein, carbohydrates or fat. There are basically 3 types of digestive enzymes and they are: proteases, which digest protein, lipases, which digest fat, and amylases, which digest carbohydrates. These 3 main groups of digestive enzymes are produced in our mouth, stomach, liver, pancreas and intestines, but they are also available in fresh foods like fruits and vegetables.

In the complicated process of digestion, food has to be processed step by step at every stage, moving from one stage to another before digestion can be completed. For example, the digestion of complex carbohydrates starts in the mouth through the production of ptyalin, which is an amylase. Once treated with ptyalin, complex carbohydrates move from the stomach to the small intestine in semi-digested form, ready to be digested further by different enzymes in the small intestine. If complex carbohydrates do not get properly treated by ptyalin, due to insufficient chewing for example, they will move into the small intestine in a form that cannot successfully be further digested, which will likely cause reactions such as indigestion, bloating, gas, diarrhoea and even cancer in the long run. Undigested food in our body causes an accumulation of bacteria that then further causes putrefaction and creates gas. This example of undigested carbohydrates causing problems in the later stages of digestion applies to proteins, fats and fibre as well. The lack of production of just one enzyme in the stomach for example, will heavily compromise protein digestion in the small intestine. All of this points strongly to the importance of digestive enzymes in every part of the digestive system. If even one of the enzymes in the very delicate process of digestion is lacking, the whole process and absorption level can be jeopardized.

To be produced in sufficient amounts, enzymes also require the presence of other substances called co-enzymes and co-factors. Co-enzymes are usually B vitamins (other vitamins, like vitamin C, also help enzymatic actions) which participate in the activation of the enzymes themselves. Co-factors are substances necessary for the functions of enzymes. Some co-factors are minerals such as zinc, calcium, magnesium and copper.

Digestive enzymes begin their action in the mouth and then continue in the small and large intestine in order to further break the food down and make it possible to assimilate. Ptyalin is the first enzyme produced by salivary glands in the mouth and its job is to break down carbohydrates and prepare them for further digestion in the stomach and small intestine. Once food reaches the stomach, the main organ responsible for the digestion of proteins, other enzymes such as pepsin, rennin and hydrochloric acid go to work.

The next stage of digestion occurs in the small intestine as food which has been digested to a certain degree in the stomach gets released into the small intestine, where it is called chyme. The small intestine is 23 feet long and is where the majority of digestion and the absorption of proteins, fats and carbohydrates takes place. The small intestine has 3 parts: the duodenum, the jejunum and the ileum. In the first part of the small intestine, the duodenum, bile is secreted from the liver and pancreatic enzymes continue digestion and absorption. In the jejunum, more enzymes such as trypsin, maltase and nuclease are secreted.

The large intestine is the last part of the digestive system and is about 5 feet long. By the time digested food reaches the large intestine, most of the nutrients have been absorbed in the small intestine; the major process that occurs in the large intestine is the absorption of water and elimination of any undigested food.

Enzyme Suppressors

Enzymes can only work properly in their natural environment. If they are exposed to different or unnatural conditions they will be eliminated and unable to act properly. The conditions that can disable enzymatic activity are either chemical or related to temperature. For me, preserving the life-boosting enzymes in the food that we eat is the ultimate art of preparing food. All that we have been offered in cookbooks so far is the art of denaturalizing the enzymes in our food and converting live food into dead food. That dead food is the major cause of our health reality, or more accurately, health misery. Dead food is nothing but a burden of empty calories and a hard task for the body to cope with. The fewer enzymes contained in the food you consume, the more enzymes need to be produced by the liver, pancreas and other organs, and the more that individual organs become involved in enzyme production, the less life energy is left for the body, leading to lowered immunity. The more that the food we eat contains active enzymes, the less organ production of enzymes is required, hence stronger immunity. Now that we have identified enzymes in food as critical immunity boosters, it should not be difficult to understand why it is so important to eat fresh and raw foods.

Let's have a look now at some of the most common processes that destroy enzymes and lead to dead food. Unfortunately, established and common practices of cooking and preserving food have silently created the indirect causes of most of our chronic diseases today. Although food preservation has enabled better and longer access to food throughout the year for a majority of the population, this hasn't been achieved without a price.

The most common process of preparing food is through cooking. Since the discovery of fire, humans have enjoyed the pleasure of eating cooked food, firstly meat, and then afterwards everything else. After millions of years of evolving around raw food, humans ventured into a new direction, substituting raw and fresh food with cooked food. Cooked food has become the subject of a new art adopted by every single culture today: the art of cookery. Hundreds, if not thousands, of cookbooks are being written by celebrity chefs, showbiz celebrities and others, bombarding us with new ideas all the time and all competing in the art of killing food. By adding different spices, seasonings, aromas, tonnes of salt and sugar, and endlessly exposing food to temperatures higher than 100 degrees C, they all promote "delicious" edibles that hardly resemble the natural foods which we evolved around and responded to with strong immunity and great health. New cheap foods have offered us great "taste" but also a lot of suffering. Cooking disables all the enzymes, producing dead food.

But there are also other processes in food preservation that can eliminate enzymes from the food, creating more bad health consequences. Those processes are: drying, freezing, bleaching, canning, milling and refining. All of these processes simply deplete food of the enzymes, co-enzymes, co-factors, fibre and water that is necessary for chemical reactions to occur. All that is preserved are empty calories, mainly in the form of carbohydrates, fats and some protein, but totally denatured. When that food is eaten it creates a completely different situation within the body compared to natural fresh food. The body has to work much harder in order to recognize the components of preserved foods and all the unnatural chemicals found in that kind of food, and has to produce many different enzymes in order to break down all those components. That huge amount of work and effort puts extra strain on the enzyme producers, such as the pancreas, liver and stomach. Those organs, when overstressed for a period of time, will literally start giving up! Indigestion, gastritis, ulcers, glucose intolerance, insulin resistance, anaemia, diabetes, liver disorders, colon cancer; these are just some of the problems that will result as consequences of eating processed, enzyme-free, dead food over a long period of time.

Other enzyme inhibitors such as alcohol, nicotine and drugs are present in the daily lives of many people and become unhealthy habits over time. Consumption of these inhibitors must also be taken into consideration when looking at lifestyle habits affecting our health and well being.

Fresh fruits and vegetables

For everyone who simply wants to live a healthy life, free of all the troubles, fears, discomforts, disappointments and disruptions that illness brings, eating healthily is a must. Nothing will enhance immunity more than healthy eating. Regular exercise will help a lot, but eating the right food is still the single most powerful factor in preserving health, strengthening immunity and improving the quality of life.

Eating fresh fruits and vegetables is the best way to start any healthy diet. Adding healthy oils, raw nuts, fish and lean meats is the next step, although we have to cook certain foods such as meat and fish to a certain degree, to make sure that what we eat is bacteriologically safe.

Unfortunately modern livestock also suffers the same fate as humans in terms of eating and physical activity. The livestock that we eat today is not free to run in nature and graze on healthy, enzyme-rich plants. Instead, they are bred and slaughtered in a very limited space and time, whilst at the same time fed with unnatural food that for them, natural herbivores, is often made of their own body parts, fish, or grains, all of which have never been present before in their natural diets! Herbivores were not created to eat grains, which are their staple food in commercial farms! Nor were they intended to eat meat and bones! So it's no wonder that the animals that we eat suffer from so many diseases and also have to be treated with so many chemicals (antibiotics) in order to be edible. All of these things are good reasons for us to make sure that the meat we eat today is cooked or exposed to high temperatures that will kill bacteria and potentially harmful chemicals.

The benefits of eating fresh fruits and vegetables are vast. Not only do they bring with them an abundance of different enzymes, antioxidants, anti-carcinogens, vitamins, minerals, and necessary fibre, but they also bring a lot of bulk with very few calories. The low caloric density and high enzymatic presence in fresh fruit and vegetables literally make them super foods!

Enzyme-rich food is always full of fibre, which is so important for the movement of food though the digestive tract and the peristaltic action, which ensures that the food passes through in the right sequences, without accumulating and disintegrating in certain parts of the digestive tract. Fibre is also known to lower cholesterol levels, which improves cardiovascular health.

High levels of enzymes in our food also help in digesting the protein, fat and carbohydrates that we eat on a daily basis. The influence of the enzymes from the food that we eat also manifests itself in less strain on the organs that produce enzymes, preserving them and therefore strengthening immunity at the same time. So not only can we gain a healthier life from eating enzyme-rich food, but also a longer and more productive life!

The bottom line

- Enzymes are protein-based chemicals that control all metabolic processes in the body.
- Enzymes are involved in the digestion of food, strengthening of the immune system, energy transfers in the body and many other essential processes.
- Enzymes are naturally found in fresh foods such as fruit, vegetables, fish and meat.
- Food processing such as chemical treatments, exposure to very high or very low temperatures and drying deactivates (eliminates) enzymes.
- Apart from food processing, there are other enzyme suppressants such as nicotine, alcohol and drugs that can deplete enzymes.
- Food that is poor in enzymes is a big burden for our digestive system; a lot of energy is needed for production of many enzymes in high quantities, leading to lowered immunity.
- There are three basic groups of digestive enzymes: proteases that digest proteins, lipases that digest fats and amylases that digest carbohydrates.
- Diets rich in fresh fruit, vegetables, raw fish and meat (that has to be cooked to be bacteriologically safe) provide many different enzymes which help to maintain good health and strengthen our immune systems.

Protein Supplements

Protein supplements definitely deserve a whole chapter on their own. Protein powders and amino acids in tablet or capsule form have taken the supplement world by storm. They have become so common in the daily diets of millions of people around the world that one would have to ask: are they still supplements or have they become foods nowadays?

In the early seventies, when the hysteria about protein powders first started, protein powders were taken very seriously. They were seen as some sort of revolutionary supplement that would mysteriously and in record time increase muscle tissue and help people get rid of all the extra body fat that they had accumulated around their bellies. What nobody wanted to admit or accept back then was that protein powders were being used as a food replacement. Protein powders in those days were simply surrounded by mystical powers that promised to deliver quick and massive changes in record time. And until now, protein powders have preserved that mystical power and the impression that they can somehow be the main method of losing fat and increasing muscle tissue.

My own experience with protein powders from my early days of bodybuilding would certainly be the best example of protein powders' almost "hypnotising" effect. I was about 16 years old when I came across my first protein powder. Endorsed by the king of bodybuilding himself, Arnold Schwarzenegger, it was imported from Germany and was chocolate flavoured, delivering an amazing promise to increase

lean muscle mass in just a matter of days. This claim was supported
by a photo of a massive muscular body, which was needed to convince people back then. Although I didn't get my new muscles within "just days" and didn't experience more than constant indigestion
and a bloated gut, I still continued to drink that protein shake and
awaited the great results "once I got used to the ultimately perfect
product". In my mind it wasn't the protein powder that was to blame
for my lack of results, but my inability to adapt to that phenomenal
product! My later experience with numerous different protein powders proved that the protein products which appeared in the seventies
were made of very poor quality ingredients, which caused all kinds
of digestive problems without any results. Protein supplements in
the eighties were much better, made of better ingredients that were
much easier to digest and even gave considerable results. The problem that I didn't notice then was that protein supplements had slowly
but surely become my main food source, whilst real food became
just a supplement to my diet! I had become just another victim of
the powerful advertising campaigns of the protein supplement industry through the bodybuilding media.

Protein supplements can only be used as such, as supplements (if
needed at all), and they must not become a substitute for real food.
In no way can protein powder compete with real food. Protein powders should be used only in order to boost protein intake in individuals who, for one reason or another, have difficulties eating enough
protein-rich food. I know many people who literally live on protein
powders, eating real food only occasionally! Convenience is the
major reason for this. Protein shakes are easily and quickly made,
taste good, and can be consumed in only a minute or two. It is much
easier and faster to drink protein than to eat protein, and preparing
protein shakes takes much less time than preparing a healthy protein

meal. Occasionally you can use the convenience factor in order to make sure that you don't miss a meal or go for the wrong type of food when hungry. If there is no time to eat, or there is no good choice of food for your meal, a protein shake may do the job - but that should only be done once in a while. Drinking protein shakes instead of having proper meals should never become a habit.

As hard as protein manufacturers may try, they will never be able to create a perfect substitute for natural food containing the right combination and ratio of essential macronutrients, accompanied by selected vitamins, minerals, trace elements and enzymes. To make it worse for the protein powder approach, all the ingredients in natural foods are unprocessed; natural foods don't contain artificial sweeteners, colours or flavours, and their minerals and trace elements are colloidal (100% absorbable). If we take a closer look at the contents of protein powders, we find that they are made from highly processed milk or egg proteins, artificial sweeteners, artificial colours, artificial aromas, and have no enzymes (or a few processed ones). So in my opinion, protein powders have become the most successful artificial food, or fake food. Always bear that in mind when you decide to have a protein shake. While you may indulge in them occasionally for temporary lack of other protein or as a supplement, they should definitely not be over-relied upon as a regular component of your diet or as a main meal.

Protein shakes have another disadvantage when it comes to fat loss and that is the lack of thermic effect. Natural food, because of its texture (composed of fibre, fat, protein, carbohydrates and other ingredients in perfect balance), causes the body to slightly increase heat production and use a substantial amount of energy for digestion. Increased heat production burns fat and the heat increases after every meal. This is the reason why 5 - 6 meals composed of natural food will make you much leaner than 2 - 3 meals or protein shakes. Protein shakes in contrast, being liquid, very smooth, having no fibre content and often hydrolysed (pre-digested), need much less energy for digestion and therefore don't burn enough calories and don't increase our resting metabolism like natural food meals do. So, if you are trying to get in shape by losing some body fat, make sure that your meals are composed of low calorie natural foods full of fibre and other necessary ingredients.

Protein powders are made of different ingredients: they are either made from the milk protein casein, or from egg protein, soy protein or whey protein. Some manufacturers use one ingredient whilst others combine them in different proportions. Whatever the combination of main protein ingredients in the particular protein powder may be, the aim is always to increase the level of absorption. Manufacturers always make different claims promising that the ingredients that they use in specific combinations will guarantee maximal absorption. The fact is that nobody can really be sure how much protein from protein powders we actually do absorb. The experience of many athletes has shown that protein powders do get absorbed and do work in combination with healthy foods, but how much of these particular products we really absorb is difficult to say.

The technology that is used in protein supplement production today is much more advanced than in the seventies when production started. Instead of powdered milk mixed with soy protein from back then, today we have a new generation of protein products made of high quality whey protein, caseins, and enriched with all necessary minerals, vitamins and enzymes, with a much higher absorption rate than products of the past.

Casein and Whey

The major difference between protein powders which has recently emerged is the difference between "slow" and "fast" proteins. Slow absorbing proteins are the ones that get digested more slowly while fast absorbing proteins get digested and absorbed quickly into the muscle tissue. There are "experts" who claim that slow absorbing proteins are better for you, but also "experts" who will try to convince you that faster absorbed proteins are better. Depending on which "clan" they belong to, different experts will try to convince you to buy one product or another.

Slow absorbing protein powders are the ones made predominantly from casein, which is the main protein in milk. Casein resembles real food more than other types of milk protein because it contains polypeptides, protein molecules that are made from many different amino acids, which are what most of the other proteins are made of. Because polypeptides have to be digested (broken down into single amino acids, dipeptides and tripeptides) in order to be absorbed, they will take more time to be utilised and hence casein is considered a slow absorbing protein.

Fast absorbing proteins are the ones made mainly from whey protein, which are much higher in dipeptides and tripeptides than casein. This specific molecular structure enables whey protein to be digested very quickly because dipeptides and tripeptides need no further digestion and breaking down in order to be absorbed efficiently by the body. So the question that arises is: who would benefit more from casein and who would benefit more from whey protein?

Since casein is a more complex protein, composed of polypeptides, it takes longer to be digested and protein shakes made wholly or mainly from casein are more like a meal. It would take 2 - 3 hours before you would be ready to eat again after having a casein protein shake. So if you, for any reason, want to replace your meal with a protein shake, a casein-based shake would be a better choice. In addition, our digestive system did evolve around complex protein structures, which would suggest that casein protein should be the first choice.

So what are the benefits of taking whey protein-based shakes? Whey hydrolysate is rich in dipeptides and tripeptides and is absorbed much more quickly than casein, whilst also being very rich with branched-chain amino acids known as BCAA. This can be an advantage for people who are involved in intense sports where strength and muscle size matter. Whey hydrolysate (better than whey isolate because of higher absorption rates along with less fat and lactose) taken before and after intense training sessions (boxing, sprinting, swimming, resistance training, etc.) provides the body with all the amino acids necessary to protect and replace burned muscle proteins. In some cases, the combination of casein and whey protein powders at different times of the day is the best choice.

The content of protein in a shake should be between 30 and 50 grams depending on important factors such are age, gender, lean body weight, training intensity, etc. Over-stuffing yourself with more than that amount will simply put extra stress on the body to digest and absorb the ingested protein, even lowering the amount of protein that can be absorbed in a particular meal (protein shake). Anything more than enough will never be as good as enough. Always blend your shakes with water and juices, not milk. Adding fresh fruit and/or flax seed oil in your shakes can help the digestion of protein and improve absorption. Up to 5 grams of glutamine can also be added into the shakes in order to satisfy the increased demand for it after intense training sessions.

I always prefer protein shakes to protein bars for a very good reason. Being the best fake food available, protein shakes resemble natural foods much more since they are composed of around 20% dry matter and 80% water (similar to meat or fish). This helps the body recognise them more as food, as opposed to protein bars which are almost devoid of water and much higher in dry matter at 70-80%.

Amino acids

Amino acids are the building blocks of protein. In order to be digested, protein has to first be broken down in smaller components (amino acids) so that it can be absorbed. There are 22 amino acids in total, but only 8 of them are ones that the body cannot produce and these are referred to as essential amino acids. Since the body can't produce them, they have to be taken in via the food that we eat. If the protein that we eat contains all of the essential amino acids it's called a complete protein and can be absorbed completely (or at a very high rate). Complete proteins allow faster and better tissue regeneration, better immunity and better overall heath. The sources of complete proteins are the animal proteins such as meat, fish, eggs, milk products, etc. Protein that comes from plants doesn't have all the essential amino acids, and these are referred to as incomplete proteins. Long-term consumption of incomplete proteins causes many different conditions because of the lack of some essential amino acids, disturbing the body's extremely important protein metabolism. For example, grains are very low in lysine whilst legumes lack methionine. For optimal protein absorption and all the benefits that come with it, complete proteins have to be eaten in adequate amounts several times per day, since we cannot store protein in the same way that we can store fat and carbohydrates.

In an attempt to produce protein products that deliver the most effective and optimal absorption levels, manufacturers have come up with an answer by offering amino acid supplements. Amino acid products are another type of protein supplement that have been used by many people with digestive problems, and those involved in sports and resistance training in order to increase muscle tissue recovery and muscle growth.

Amino acid supplements may come in the form of a powder, liquid, capsules or tablets, and fall into three categories. The first category is made up of the amino acid products that contain all 22 acids. These products are nothing but the whole protein delivered in tablet form. If they are all present together in the same product they will lead to the same results as protein powder which contains the same amount and number of amino acids. They should be viewed as basically the same as protein powders on their own.

The second category represents the products that contain only single amino acids. There are some amino acids that have been marketed by the manufacturers as acids that can improve sleep, stimulate higher growth hormone production or have some very specific effect on a particular biochemical process in the body. A well-promoted single amino acid is tryptophan which allegedly improves sleep patterns and relaxation. Other very popular amino acids that are sold separately include arginine, lysine and ornithine. It has been claimed that these amino acids can increase production of a "magic" growth

hormone responsible for organ repair, fat burning, muscle building and the overall rejuvenation process. Unfortunately, scientific
research hasn't proven any significant amount of growth hormone
increase after taking these single amino acids in the recommended
dosages. Regular and deep sleep, high intensity resistance training
and a healthy diet are still the best natural ways to optimise growth
hormone production.

Glutamine is another very popular amino acid sold separately. Being
the most abundant amino acid in the skeletal muscles, glutamine is
also the amino acid that is most used in everyday intense training
regimes. Therefore, as advertised by amino acids manufacturers,
glutamine is the most important single amino acid which should be
taken immediately after intense training sessions in order to replace
the glutamine that has been used by the heavy muscle contractions
that occur during resistance training.

In the third category belong the amino acid products that are made
up of two or three amino acids together. By far the most popular
in this group are the amino acids known as branched-chain amino
acids or BCAA. They are composed of three amino acids: leacine,
isoleucine and valine. BCAA are especially popular among athletes
who are involved in intense sports. As well as carbohydrates and fat,
protein is a source of energy relied upon during sport activities. The
amino acids in the muscle tissue that get used the most are actually
leucine, isoleucine and valine or BCAA. Being so important for
muscle tissue, BCAA represents the bulk of amino acids (50 - 90 %)
absorbed in the first three hours after a protein meal! Taking BCAA
supplements before and after exercise offers a solution of sparing
BCAA during the exercise and then replacing them quickly after the
training session. The suggested daily amount of BCAA tops 10 000

mg, while an amount of 4 000 mg is a more conservative approach. The best time to take BCAA is before and after exercise.

There are also amino acids that belong to this group called peptide-bonded amino acids. Amino acids work best when they are paired in groups of two or three amino acids together, called dipeptides and tripeptides. Peptide-bonded amino acids are more easily absorbed than single amino acids because of the body's evolutionary patterns. The recommended daily amount for peptide-bonded amino acids is around 10 000 to 12 000 mg daily, divided in 3 - 4 doses after meals.

Amino acids are one of the most trusted types of products in the supplement world. Promising great results with just a few tablets taken daily, amino acids have established a very strong position in the supplement shopping list of consumers looking to achieve great results with minimum effort, whether it be better health in general, fat loss or gaining a few pounds of new muscle.

Amino acid products that contain all the amino acids are nothing but encapsulated protein powder. If you believe that the human body has been created in order to digest protein in the form of tablets that have been heavily processed, you will need a lot of luck with that approach. The human digestive system still absorbs protein best when it comes from natural protein sources such as meat, fish, eggs, etc. Spend your money wisely. Single amino acids like arginine and ornithine, which have been advertised as great growth hormone promoters, do very little to increase this most famous hormone. Any increase in growth hormone caused by an intake of these single amino acids is always questionable. If you are looking to increase growth hormone production it's better to concentrate on a GH-promoting regimen: high intensity resistance training and adequate sleep. This advice will definitely save you a lot of money and broken dreams. When it comes to branched-chain amino acids or BCAA serious athletes, especially bodybuilders, have used them religiously. From my own experience, and the experience of many professional athletes that I have worked with, BCAA were never as essential as they have been promoted to be. I believe that BCAA taken before and after training in high amounts (3 - 4 grams) may benefit athletes who don't take enough protein in their daily diet or don't take whey protein before and after training sessions, but if you eat enough high quality protein at intervals during the day then you will completely satisfy your need for BCAA during and after intense training sessions. Whey protein powders are another cheaper option; however, eating enough natural food is definitely the best option.

Putting all the previously mentioned pros and cons together brings me to the conclusion that the best choice for long term improvement in sports, fat loss, muscle growth and improved health is to eat enough fresh high quality foods, as nature intended us to. I was hugely surprised when I discovered in my early days in sports that top professional bodybuilders — for example the same ones that have been advertising and endorsing many different supplements like protein powders, hormone enhancers, amino acids and other similar products — were the same ones who were only eating natural foods and nothing else! Some of them were eating a lot of red meat, others lots of chicken, whilst some were combining meat, chicken and fish. Fresh vegetables and fruit also played a major part in their diet. They were simply giving the body the best food available after intense resistance training sessions. Whilst vitamins and minerals did play their role in the diets of those top athletes, protein powders and amino acids did not play important roles.

After years of taking so many different protein powders and amino acids (single, peptide-bonded, BCAA and others) it wasn't easy for me to give these up and try training and aiming for top results by relying only on natural foods – it was actually incomprehensible! But I also couldn't resist the challenge to try something that was so compelling at the same time. Eventually I tried it; I started eating more natural food, eating more often and incorporating more fresh vegetables in my diet than ever before. So what were the results? After 2 - 3 weeks I became much firmer, I wasn't bloated at all, and had more energy than ever before. Soon after that, I experienced a surge in my strength and my muscle size started improving. Although I didn't stop drinking protein shakes, food soon became my dominant source of protein, fat and carbohydrates. Now, protein shakes are there just to fill the gap and I only use them occasionally as a matter of convenience.

I hope my experience will help you draw your own conclusions when it comes to these heavily processed and denatured products which make the immensely profitable supplement industry a reality of our time. Remember that we have evolved around natural foods, and our digestive system performs with the highest efficiency only when we stick to the foods that our bodies best recognize because of millions of years of evolution. Anything processed, denatured, concentrated, dehydrated, or frozen will not be recognized by the body as food, and in many instances will be treated as an outside invader rather than as necessary food. Food in the form of pills or powders is definitely not the food that our physiology prefers although, for the sake of convenience, we can make exceptions - as long as they don't become part of our regular eating habits.

The bottom line

- All protein supplements are made from real food. Using different food processing technologies, protein is extracted from real food and is then delivered in powder or tablet form.
- The main protein supplements are protein powders and amino acids in tablet or capsule form.
- Many people over-estimate the importance of protein supplements and substitute them for real food.
- Protein supplements are only supplements, they are not real food and they will never be as good as real food.
- In order to increase absorption rates to try to match those of real food, protein supplements are usually enriched with different minerals, vitamins and digestive enzymes.
- The biggest advantage of protein supplements over real food is in the convenience factor. Protein shakes are made easily and quickly, and they can also taste good.
- Absorption of protein supplements and their total effect on the metabolic processes in the body will never be as high as from natural food.
- The major components of protein powders are casein and whey, two different proteins extracted from milk.
- Whey protein is much more easily absorbed then casein, making it a fast protein which is more beneficial after high intensity training sessions because of its rapid absorption. Casein is digested more slowly, providing a constant flow of amino acids over a longer period of time. Casein is much more efficient when consumed as the last protein intake of the day

Other Supplements

Protein powders and amino acids remain the most popular, most advertised and best-selling food supplements in an industry that turns out over $20 billion in the USA every year, but they are not the only supplements on the market. Since we all want to achieve as much as possible with as little effort as possible, supplements perfectly fit into that general lifestyle approach, and there are many other supplements that attract the attention of ordinary folk as well as fitness enthusiasts and athletes all over the world. With minimal effort and a few pills per day, we hope to achieve great health, sexual vigour, high energy levels, lots of muscles and low levels of body fat. All of this is approved and supported by a highly developed marketing industry geared towards followers of a pill culture.

There are hundreds of different products out there that are considered supplements and ergogenics, and many of them have already secured huge market shares. Millions of people around the globe gobble handfuls of different supplement pills every morning, hoping that by taking them they will escape the perils of a poor lifestyle, improper eating and physical inactivity. The results that millions of people expect from their favourite supplements range from lower cholesterol levels, lower blood pressure, improved circulation, improved memory, increased testosterone production, overcoming depression, higher energy, fat loss and muscle growth. It is difficult, living in this modern pill culture age, to ignore the promise that pills seem to give us, where they are thought of as the most authoritative, trustworthy and reliable friend who is always available, whenever and however much we need them. The promise of health, happiness and vigour in the form of a pill is difficult to turn down!

Unfortunately, supplements have taken over healthy eating, regular exercise and healthy lifestyles in general by simply promising the same benefits with much less effort. Just ask yourself how many people you know who exercise regularly and follow a healthy diet vs. how many people you know that take a whole range of supplements and sound like experts from the homeopathic or supplement industry? How many times have you heard about the amazing affects of one supplement or another that can lower your blood pressure or make you lose fat whilst still eating anything you want? And how many times have you heard from people you know who have lost a lot of body fat since they started exercising on a daily basis and started following a healthy diet? I bet that the supplement proponents constitute the majority of people that you know and that supplements are winning the battle when it comes to choosing the tools for a healthier and happier life.

Although some supplements do positively alter our biochemistry and bring about beneficial physiological changes, the question that we should ask is: are they really so effective that the changes they bring about are significant enough to deliver on what they promise?

Let's now have a look at the leading products in the supplement world, the most popular and heavily marketed supplements, and see what they offer. This list includes glucosamine sulfate, ginkgo biloba, St. John's wort, ginseng, CoQ10, melatonin, garlic, echinacea, saw palmetto, creatine, HMB, etc.

Glucosamine Sulfate

With staggering sales topping $280 million in the USA every year, glucosamine sulfate is the undisputed king of the general supplements market. But before we look at the claims that manufacturers of this wonder supplement promise to the public, let's first look at the nature of this substance.

Glucosamine is a natural substance that is produced by the body and helps in the production of lubricants in the joints, keeping them supple. It is also involved in the production of structural components of joint cartilage. With age, the body loses the ability to produce sufficient amounts of glucosamine, causing degeneration of the joints which further causes damage to cartilage. If we remind ourselves and agree that the majority of people in the developed world over the age of 50 are overweight, it wouldn't be difficult to understand that extra weight puts more pressure on the joints, therefore causing joint deformation. Other factors that increase the potential risk for joint damage are poor nutrition (which deprives the body of the essential macro- and micro-elements necessary for joint and cartilage repair), inactivity (which slows down metabolic efficiency and demand for strong connective tissues and joints), and extreme over-training in different sports (which puts tremendous pressure on the joints and cartilage).

Glucosamine sulfate is the most readily absorbed form of glucosamine in the body and, taken for longer periods of time in dosages of up to 1 500 mg per day, may offer prevention of and a potential cure for cartilage problems and also for joint repair.

Ginkgo Biloba

Ginkgo biloba, or simply ginkgo, has been around for centuries. Chinese herbal medicine has been using ginkgo leaves and seeds for centuries in preventing and curing many different health problems. Today's modern preventative medicine now relies more on ginkgo extract, which is more potent because it provides a concentrate of the major components in ginkgo that are found to have profound effects on human health: flavonoids (quercentin and rutin) and terpenoids (ginkgolides). While flavonoids have a potent antioxidant effect, protecting heart muscles, nerves and blood vessels, terpenoids improve blood flow by dilating blood vessels and reducing the stickiness of blood platelets.

Ginkgo biloba's popularity has helped achieve annual sales of $145 million in the USA alone! Ginkgo is claimed to improve circulatory disorders and enhance memory. By enhancing memory, ginkgo is also believed to improve the learning process, and general improvements in daily living and social behaviours have also been attributed to this supplement. Ginkgo is also used to combat asthma, depression, headaches and high blood pressure. It's often given to help reduce the side effects of menopause and osteoporosis, and decrease the risk of cardiovascular diseases. The recommended daily amount is 120 mg taken in 2-3 equally divided doses.

St. John's Wort

The third most popular commercial supplement, by all market indications, is St. John's wort. Used for many years, this supplement is believed to deliver a remedy for mild depression, sleep disturbances and anxiety. Some research suggests that St. John's wort raises the body's levels of serotonin and dopamine, and this helps to boost morale and one's overall mood.

St. John's wort has become a favourite supplement for people suffering from mild depression. Dosages of 900 mg per day taken in three equal amounts of 300 mg have been reported to benefit those who suffer from depression. More scientific research is needed, however, to prove the real effectiveness of St. John's wort.

Ginseng

Used by Chinese medicine for thousands of years, ginseng has been attributed with providing increased longevity and vitality. Whilst the aging process is sped up by decreased functions of the nervous system, endocrine system and lowered immunity, components found in ginseng have been shown to improve the functions of these systems and even bring them closer to a normal level. Some research has shown that saponins (substances found in ginseng) stimulate the immune response of the body, and also revitalize the functions and tissues of internal organs such as the liver and kidneys.

In experiments with elderly people, ginseng has increased the activity of lymphocytes, whilst in animals, ginseng has proven to prolong life span, improve motor activity and increase the production of antibodies. Ginseng has also benefited in popularity largely because of claims that it can increase stamina and offer a higher quality of life. Some research has shown a slight increase in alertness, improved relaxation and appetite in people who regularly take ginseng extract. Other experiments, however, have not shown significant improvement or increased endurance in athletes and physically active people who take ginseng supplements.

Although there are indications that the saponins in ginseng trigger some biochemical processes in the body, more research is needed on human subjects, since most of the research to date has only been conducted on animals.

Melatonin

Melatonin is a hormone produced by the pineal gland from the amino acid tryptophan. This is a light-sensitive hormone, manufactured by the body in the absence of light. It is believed that melatonin may control the body's internal clock and also our sleep cycle. Melatonin production decreases with age, and this may be the reason for the lack of sleep or reduced need for sleep in elderly people.

Melatonin is mainly used in order to induce sleep, to help people with sleeping difficulties, and to offset the problems of jetlag. People with insomnia often look for help through melatonin supplements. Melatonin doesn't just fight insomnia, however; it is also claimed to strengthen immunity and act as a very powerful antioxidant, scavenging free radicals to a degree that even surpasses that of the extra powerful antioxidant vitamin E! There are also claims that melatonin is a potent protector of the heart. Low levels of melatonin in the body have been associated with depression, and melatonin supplements may be beneficial in combating this. Improved longevity in animals during experiments where they were given melatonin supplements opens even more room for speculation as to the possible benefits of this very popular supplement. The recommended daily amount of melatonin supplements is 1 mg per day taken at bedtime. Melatonin should not be taken during active parts of the day.

More scientific research and research on humans is needed in order to prove the real effectiveness of melatonin supplements.

Garlic

Garlic has been used for hundreds of years as a food, and recently as a supplement to combat infections, strengthen immunity and lower cholesterol. Numerous overall health benefits have been attributed to this plant, and more recently to garlic supplements.

Garlic is thought to be a very effective antiseptic, preventing wound infections. The substance found in garlic, called allicin, is thought to be responsible for the anti-bacterial action. Another component found in garlic is ajoene, which has been found to have strong anti-fungal qualities. There are also some anti-cancer properties attributed to garlic, whilst some studies have also shown that garlic can lower blood pressure and cholesterol levels.

Although very popular as a supplement, garlic has not shown significant results in terms of overall health improvement or illness prevention. People who like to eat garlic or take garlic supplements should not expect dramatic changes if they suffer from disease or illness. Garlic can help to some degree, but it won't be enough to compete with radical lifestyle changes and medical approaches to serious health problems.

Creatine Monohydrate

Creatine monohydrate definitely stands out among the ever-popular sports supplements that are one of the most profitable niche markets. Many athletes who are looking to increase muscle size, strength, speed and endurance have used creatine. Some of them have claimed great results such as weight increases of 8 - 10 pounds in only 2 weeks! There are also reports that some athletes have dramatically increased their strength level in a very short period of time.

So what is behind the apparent success of creatine supplements? Creatine monohydrate is known to cause cell volumization, which means that it has the ability to directly draw water and other nutrients into the muscle cells, increasing muscle size and fullness. But in order for supplemental creatine to be successfully absorbed, it has to be of very high quality. High quality powdered creatine, for example, requires an extremely fine grinding procedure that results in the same molecular size of creatine that is found in natural foods and is thus easily absorbable. The biggest creatine manufacturers also claim that their products are more effective than others because they add high glycemic carbohydrates to their creatine products. The reason for this is, they claim, that the body increases insulin output immediately after consuming creatine when sugars (dextrose) are added. Insulin is the hormone produced by the pancreas that drives nutrients, including creatine monohydrate, into the muscle cells. So in the presence of the powerful hormone insulin, the chances of creatine absorption increase significantly.

The problem that I have with the above claim is that insulin, as the most powerful muscle building hormone, will always bring extra nutrients including creatine into the cells as long as its presence is sufficient. So, by including high glycemic carbohydrates in creatine drinks, it will raise insulin levels in the blood and directly increase the ability to deliver nutrients to the cells anyway. Is creatine needed there at all? Is it creatine or insulin that actually causes cell volumization? Well, this is the question that creatine manufacturers never ask.

My personal experience would not please the creatine advocates. I had the opportunity to try creatine at a time when it was not yet available on the market (it was the "best kept secret" of American athletes and I remember well the day when creatine arrived in a big plastic case direct from America). The instructions were as follows: loading for 5 days with 20 grams of creatine each day, followed by 5 grams daily during a maintenance phase. I have to admit that this was the first time in my life that I have had diarrhoea for 5 consecutive days! But still I was convinced that this was the way it was supposed to work! In the weeks that followed, apart from water retention, I didn't experience any strength gain or increase in lean muscle tissue. I don't know about the weight increase, but if there was any it must have been from the extra water I retained thanks to the creatine "magic".

Whilst insulin acts as one of the most potent cell volumizers, everyone should be aware that insulin is a double-edged sword. Insulin can dramatically increase muscle size, but can also dramatically increase fat storage in the body. Insulin is not only needed for optimal glycogen storage, muscle growth, and maintenance, but it will also divert glucose and other nutrients into the fat stores. Adding insulin to defend and justify the powers of creatine has never been the most convincing aspect of the creatine marketing strategy.

Since it is quite new on the supplement market (first offered in 1994), reatine monohydrate has definitely missed the golden age of body-building (1970-80) when people like Arnold, Frank Zane, Colombo, and others were winning competitions and displaying amazing physiques and great muscle fullness without even knowing about creatine. So if they managed to do it without creatine, the question that arises is, do we really need creatine to achieve results that don't necessarily equal those of the great bodybuilders?

The highest concentration of naturally occurring creatine is found in meat and fish. If we know that a person weighing 70 kilograms needs 2 grams of creatine daily, this can be obtained from 500 grams of meat or fish (or a combination of both) daily. A person with a lean bodyweight of 100 kilograms would need 750 grams of meat and fish daily to satisfy his daily requirement for creatine.

Half of the necessary creatine is made in the body from 3 amino acids: arginine, glycine and methionine. The other half of the body's required creatine has to be taken in through food or supple-ments. Since the previously mentioned amounts of protein sources are needed anyway to support health, muscle building and energy requirements, creatine needs can also be easily satisfied using these sources. If you add an extra 3 - 5 grams of creatine daily in the form of supplements, you will definitely experience the consequences of its spill-over effect: water retention will occur but in the wrong place! What you will experience is water retention in extra-cellular rather than in intra-cellular space! This is exactly what happens to the majority of creatine users. The only people that would benefit from creatine monohydrate supplements are people who don't eat enough meat and fish in their diet, or vegetarians who don't eat meat in any form.

There needs to be more independent scientific research conducted to establish the real effect of creatine supplements and verify all the benefits that have been claimed by creatine supplement manufacturers (muscle growth, strength increase, etc.). Most of the research into creatine and its benefits has, until now, only been conducted by the creatine supplement manufacturers.

If you eat enough fish, poultry and meat on a daily basis, you would be much better off investing your money in high quality foods and essential vitamin and mineral supplements than in products that can only benefit a certain (and rather small) percentage of the population.

The bottom line

- Whilst protein powders and amino acids still remain the best selling supplements on the market, there are many other supplements that attract millions of customers.
- The other popular supplements are glucosamine sulfate, ginkgo biloba, St. John's wort, ginseng, CoQ10, melatonin, garlic, echinacea, saw palmetto, creatine, HMB, etc.
- Although all these supplements do demonstrate some of the promised effects in laboratory settings, the question that remains is will they cause significant enough changes in the human body which will result in better health, more muscles, less body fat, and increased strength? If the selection, amount and combination of natural food is right, most of these supplements will have no significant effect.
- The most powerful effect of the above mentioned supplements is still the placebo effect.

Food Combination

Eating certain types of food in combination with others is not the best option for optimal digestion of food, absorption of nutrients and overall health. The food that we eat should only be combined with compatible food, leading to maximum digestion and absorption levels.

Unfortunately, most of the popular dishes that have muscled their way onto restaurant menus and dining tables involve combinations of foods that don't go together well, and therefore lead to digestive problems. Digestive problems later lead to deteriorated health in the form of allergies, heartburn, gastritis, ulcers, water retention and others. The most popular food combinations of everyday meals are, for example, steak and potatoes, chicken and rice, ham sandwiches (bread with ham), oats with milk, eggs on toast and so on. So let's have a look at what makes these food combinations difficult to digest and ultimately poor choices for overall health.

In order to be digested, protein has to be exposed to an acidic environment. Hydrochloric acid and pepsin are the substances in the stomach that digest protein. Once protein enters the stomach, these acidic juices are released and start digesting protein into smaller particles, called peptides. Peptides then get digested by peptidase enzymes, that break them down further into individual amino acids so that they can be ready for absorption. The protein that we eat can only be absorbed at the smallest particle level: amino acids. Protein-rich food spends at least 3 hours in the stomach undergoing digestion before it moves out into the small intestine.

When it comes to carbohydrate digestion, things start differently as soon carbohydrates enter the mouth. Once we start chewing starchy carbohydrates such as bread, pasta, rice, potatoes, etc., saliva glands in the mouth secrete the enzyme amylase, which starts digesting the starches before we swallow. When the food then enters the stomach, amylase stops working because of the acidic environment and digestion of the food only continues once again when it moves from the stomach into the small intestine, where more amylase is produced to complete the carbohydrates' digestion.

Fats and oils are digested slowly and mainly in the intestines by the lipase enzymes and bile, and they do not interfere much with the digestion of starch and carbohydrates. But a problem arises when you eat protein and carbohydrates together in the same meal. Whilst protein requires an acidic environment for its digestion, carbohydrates (or more precisely starches) require an alkaline or pH neutral environment in which to be digested properly. When proteins and starches enter the stomach together, the acid environment interferes with the starches by keeping them intact in the stomach for hours where they start fermenting. So when you eat chicken and rice in the same meal, for example, the rice starts fermenting in the stomach while waiting for the chicken to be digested. This will happen every time you eat a combination of protein and starches in the same meal. The basic rule then should be to avoid eating these two food groups together whenever possible.

You might wonder why nature didn't work this problem out when protein and starch represent the bulk of most of the meals that we commonly eat? The question is understandable, but the problem is that we only recently started eating this combination of food. For most of our evolution, for 4 million years up until the discovery of agriculture some 10 000 years ago, humans often only had a choice of eating either protein and fat on its own, in the form of meat and seafood, or carbohydrates on their own in the form of fruits and vegetables. Since grains didn't exist for 99.75% of our evolution, we didn't really have enough time to adapt to this new food, and especially to the combination of starches and protein together in the same meal.

We have perfectly adapted to the foods that we have evolved around and to the way in which we eat them. Humans have mainly eaten one single type of food at a time (per single meal) for most of our evolution. For example, meat was eaten on its own after hunting and fruits were eaten on their own when picked. Even today, tribes that live in remote regions of the world and who have preserved their traditional ways of living like hunters and gatherers always eat a single type of food per meal! Our ancestors didn't preserve food and keep it stored for weeks or months. Food was eaten on the spot and most likely in a hurry before other predators arrived. It is hard to imagine that our ancestors had combined foods like meat and vegetables or fruit in the same meal. This way of eating, the one that we have evolved around, allows the body to work at its best — a single food or combination of foods (meat and vegetables) in a single meal. Once you put grains (rice, pasta, bread…) and potatoes in the same meal with protein, digestive difficulties will occur.

Foods that are compatible with protein in the same meal include most vegetables, fats and acid fruits, since they all need either an acid or neutral environment for digestion. Starchy foods can be eaten together with vegetables, fats and some dried fruits.

It is important to mention that fruits are best eaten on their own, either about half an hour before a meal or between meals as a snack. Fruit sugar will quickly ferment in an acidic environment whilst waiting for protein to be digested, if eaten together. Fermented sugar will cause bloating and disturb the rest of digestion in the small intestine. Eaten on its own, fruit will be quickly digested whilst most of the sugars from the fruit will be absorbed directly by the liver without causing a sudden surge in insulin. Once again, the reasons for this process were formed during our evolution when our ancestors couldn't wait to eat or bother with food combining. They would eat as much fruit as they could whenever they could find it. Fruit is a seasonal gift in a natural environment (without freezers and big supermarkets) and was most likely eaten on its own. As our digestive system still treats fruit the same as it has for millions of years, the best option is to eat fruit on its own.

Combining food improperly doesn't only cause an upset stomach and indigestion; the consequences of incorrect food combining over a long period of time can be much more serious. Conditions such as water retention which leads to hypertension are common symptoms of improper food combining. Heartburn, allergies, headaches, weight gain and other undesirable consequences can also cause many other health problems, all of which have their roots in the wrong food combinations.

Whilst incorrect food combining affects everyone simply because of the basic laws of chemistry - acid (acidic environment) and base (alkaline environment) are incompatible and neutralise each other — the people who are most seriously affected by incorrect food combinations are the elderly. With increased age we produce fewer enzymes for digestion and less hydrochloric acid; therefore in old age it is much more difficult for the body to deal with digestive disturbances caused by incorrect food combining.

Two of the most popular recent diets which have addressed the problems of food combining and helped many people to lose extra weight and get rid of bloating and other problems are the Hay and Hollywood diets. Basically, they simply split carbohydrates and protein nto separate meals during the day so you would have, for example, 2 protein meals and 2 carbohydrate meals (or 3 each) per day.

If you need to eat complex carbohydrates for any reason, they are best digested when separated from protein and eaten on their own. Eat carbohydrates in the morning or early afternoon rather than in the evening or late at night when they are most likely to be stored as fat.

The following is a list of compatible foods:

- Protein with vegetables
- Protein with acid fruits
- Protein with fats
- Protein with fats and vegetables
- Protein with fats and acid fruits
- Starches with vegetables
- Starches with fats
- Starches with fats and vegetables
- Starches with dried fruit

To summarize the main issues of food combining, I would say that things started to go wrong the moment we abandoned our natural way of eating and introduced a completely new type of food: grains. Since then, many health problems have evolved and one of the main ones among them is improper food combination. Without grains, incompatible combinations of food wouldn't be eaten. Before grains, foods were eaten on their own and digested optimally. The improper combination of food is just a single link in the chain of unwanted consequences that have occurred since the discovery of agriculture. Nature simply never intended it this way...

The issue of bad food combining doesn't stop there. It's not just that the process of digestion gets disturbed, leading to poorer assimilation of nutrients, but also that the ideal pH balance in the blood and tissues changes depending on which foods we eat and combine. Excess amounts of acid in the blood and tissues, called acidosis, are thought to be the cause of many illnesses. So how do we get to the stage when our blood and tissues become more acidic that they should be? Too many acid producing foods in our diet and not enough foods that require an alkaline environment are the major causes of acidosis. This unwanted condition can easily happen when most of the food that we eat is made of meats, fish, bread, rise, pasta, porridge, potatoes and other acid-forming foods. In the absence of fresh fruit and vegetables which are mostly alkaline foods, our body will enter a more acidic stage.

In order to balance the alkaline and acid environment, we have to base our diets on the right proportion of acid-forming foods and foods that require an alkaline medium. According to some nutrition experts, 80% of the food that we eat should be alkaline-forming food, while 20% should come from acid-forming food. That would mean that 80% of the food that we eat daily should be composed of vegetables and fruit, and 20% should come from meats, fish, eggs and cheese. My own experience and the experiences of my clients over the last 25 years suggests that, depending on daily physical activity levels, you can derive up to 50% of your food from concentrated protein sources (meat, fish and others) and 50 % from alkaline forming foods (vegetables and fruits), maintaining good health and a high level of physical strength and stamina. So when it comes to combining food, if you stick to the 50 - 50 ratio of protein sources to fresh vegetable and fruits, you simply can't go wrong. In this scenario there will be no room for starchy foods and the incompatibility between protein and starches will be eliminated from the start. In eating fruits as snacks, separated from your main meals, you will be blessed with the perfect combination of food — either protein on its own, protein in combination with vegetables, or vegetables on their own! The perfect recipe for health!

There has been a lot said and written about food combining, but ultimately it means nothing more than the combination of protein with other macronutrients, mainly carbohydrates. But no less important than the combining of macronutrients is the nutrient interaction which happens on the micronutrient level, or between the minerals and vitamins. These essential micronutrients can also interfere with one another and fight for the receptors of the cells through which they are absorbed. The amount of every single micronutrient that we absorb daily can make the difference between good health and illness.

The interference factor occurs because nutrients do not just work alone, but in a variety of reactions and combinations with other nutrients and enzymes. When they compete with each other, certain nutrients are absorbed more than others, and nutrients which are present in greater amounts usually get absorbed better. The interference factor comes into play because some substances bind with different nutrients, causing them to pass more easily through the intestines. For example, iron is absorbed poorly without the presence of vitamin C; so if you are concerned about iron absorption, instead of supplementing your diet with iron it may be better to increase your vitamin C intake. Vitamin D is essential for calcium absorption, therefore more exposure to sunlight or supplemental vitamin D will increase the levels of calcium absorption more than by simply adding supplemental calcium. Another example of nutrient interaction is the relation between caffeine and calcium: caffeine decreases calcium absorption. Yet another example is the inhibition of vitamin E absorption by iron — these two microelements should never be taken together. If you take them, make sure that you take them separately. Selenium, on the other hand, increases the absorption of vitamin E.

Coffee and alcohol push magnesium out of the body at a much faster rate than normal. Viruses increase the requirements for zinc and B complex, whilst surgery demands a higher supply of vitamin C and calcium.

All these examples suggest that, when we think about our nutrition, we have to take into consideration not just macronutrients and their proper combination in a single meal, but also micronutrients and their interaction with each other. Since we have to supplement our diets with essential micronutrients, we have to make sure that we take them in a way that will benefit us in the best possible manner.

The bottom line

- In order to digest protein, an acidic environment is required. The first stage of protein digestion occurs in the stomach where hydrochloric acid and pepsin are produced, and continues in the small intestine where other enzymes necessary for protein digestion are secreted.

- Carbohydrates require an alkaline environment for their digestion. Digestion of starches starts in the mouth, bypasses the stomach, and continues in the small intestine where more enzymes necessary for the digestion of carbohydrates are secreted.
- Fats and oils are digested in the intestines by enzymes called lipases.
- Acidity and alkalinity neutralise each other when put together, therefore eating protein and carbohydrates in the same meal requires two different environments that are basically incompatible with each other.
- Digestion of meals that contain protein and starches will be compromised and the unwanted chemical reaction in the digestive system will cause health problems.
- Protein and starches should not be eaten in the same meal.
- Protein can be combined with vegetables in the same meal.
- Starches can be combined with vegetables in the same meal.
- Fruit should be eaten on its own, between meals

The Game of Counting Calories

Every time someone approaches me with a question regarding calories, I remember my early days of training and the then mysterious world of nutrition and calorie counting. Calorie issues always trigger questions such as: how many calories are needed to maintain basic metabolism? How much does daily calorie intake have to be reduced in order to lose body fat? How much does daily calorie intake need to be increased in order to increase lean body weight, etc...

Lack of experience in weight training and a lack of real knowledge about anatomy, physiology, nutrition and other relevant subjects have created a fear of failure and a need for quick answers in many people. It has also led us to believe that fast results and big improvements are possible in no time. This state of confusion was part of my experience as well. I remember very well the times when I bought all the books that promised answers to the most important question I wanted to answer back then: how do I get big and lean quickly? I was frantically counting calories in every single food item I ate, measuring "correct" amounts and creating "perfect" meals. I was obsessing about the perfect balance of nutrients and religiously following "scientific" outines which I had meticulously calculated. At the same ime, I was very proud of myself for having become a little scientist — everything had to be in grams and in the right proportion. In those days I wouldn't miscalculate a single calorie!

That kind of practice went on for the first 2 years of my training. At the same time I had gone from being very lean but without big muscle mass to being "big" but still carrying a lot of body fat. Throughout these experiences, I was obsessive about creating caloric strategies which I thought were supposed to give me guaranteed results. Everything was perfectly recorded and I believed that time was the only thing standing between my perfect theories and perfect end results. But after two years of intense training and even more intense mental effort, the results I achieved were not as great as I had expected. More experienced "experts" and calorie counters might suggest that my caloric intake was too low at some point, and then too high later, or that the combination of food wasn't right, and as usually happens, there are always a lot of excuses and explanations after a failure.

One thing that I had never considered back in those days was to simply follow my own instincts and react swiftly if the results were not to my satisfaction. In our modern society however, the problem is that we don't rely on our instincts until we first exhaust all of our mental tools. If my body told me that carbohydrates are not compatible with me because of water retention and fat gain, I would rather ignore the message, because it didn't agree with the theory that I had read back then! If my body told me that I needed more protein because my training sessions were more intense, I wouldn't do it simply because I was not "supposed" to do it. According to the theory I was convinced was true, eating more protein instead of the amount of carbohydrates that I had read was necessary was unthinkable! Our mathematical mind likes to see things in clear order; things should be calculated, predicted and successfully executed, such as for example in architecture, the automotive industry or any other exact sciences. As long as you work with bricks and mortar, metal and plastic, etc., a mathematical mind will be very pleased with the results which require mathematical formulas and leave no room for mistakes. This practice has brought us many benefits and comforts in modern life, and thanks to this same approach, we have technology today that has greatly improved human life. But when you apply the same philosophy to the human body, where you don't deal with bricks and mortar to support the weight of a block of flats, but with a phenomenal physiological distribution of different nutrients, vitamins, minerals, enzymes and other chemicals in order to support human life, the results are not that good.

Life, being a mystery and the most complicated subject that one can contemplate, is definitely not understandable purely through mathematical formulas. In that mystery of being, the food that we eat plays a big part, in a way transforming itself from one type of life into another. As we very well know, humans have managed to continue and to preserve life very successfully without eroding it with self-inflicted diseases for hundreds of thousands of years. Before we had discovered mathematics — counting, multiplying, measuring and of course, calories — we had enjoyed lives free of all these diseases that are now silently killing us in huge numbers. Yet still we prefer to religiously hold on to our caloric concepts — somebody's false assumptions about our own food and the same food that gives us life itself! But reality speaks for itself! As a species, we are the only one in nature that suffers from chronic diseases, weight problems and more recently from obesity. Health-wise, we are now crippled and our future doesn't look very promising. I see calorie-counting practises as a major contributor to our current health situation.

In the "caretaker" culture of the developed world, everything is expected to be taken care of and given to us without the need for our understanding or even our involvement. The food that we eat is mainly processed, some of it is ready-cooked and all that we need to do is to chew and swallow. I wouldn't be surprised if in the near future food companies started producing food that is pre-chewed!

In this "caretaking" environment, we even have solutions for eventual problems like obesity which are expected to occur. Calorie books, calorie tables, calorie calculators are readily available, and every single edible that we buy has a label showing its caloric values. So, we apparently have everything needed to eventually correct these problems and get back to our desired shape; but is it happening? Our ancestors must be laughing at us...

It is very common to see people working out in gyms carrying different booklets, brochures and diaries in which they have written all the "right" numbers of sets, reps, weights, selections of the "best" exercises, etc. But all they achieve with these is to distract themselves with totally incorrect and unnecessary calculations. I personally know a lot of little "scientific gods" who have been going to the gym for years, all armed with the latest fitness gadgets created to help measure the number of calories that they have burnt, monitor pulse rate or other games, and they are always writing or reading something while training. All that would be fine if there were some actual tangible results achieved in the process. Results? These are the only things missing...

The same situation applies when it comes to food. Calories have become the most important factors regarding food; they have replaced the importance of nutrients and other essential factors in real food. If counting calories and mathematically calculating the perfect ways of weight training were the right thing to do, would we have so many unfit people nowadays?

All these funny episodes that I often see in the gyms remind me of my own search for the truth. In those difficult days when I had to face reality and see my own illusions and lack of knowledge come crashing down around me, I remember being fascinated by seeing the best bodybuilders in the world eating their food without calculating calories and measuring the weight of every single item before eating it. They trained without writing the number of sets and reps they have done or weights they had lifted, without reading magazines and brochures before starting a set! Everything that I believed then was the best thing to do, didn't exist in the world of the bodybuilding elite at all! Their training was very intense and mainly instinctive; they would "know" or "feel" when to stop, and they didn't follow numerical systems. Food was all-natural: meat, chicken and fish and lot of vegetables. They would again "know" or "feel" when they had enough. Nobody ever measured the right weight of food for each meal, counted calories, or stopped when the pre-calculated number of calories had been eaten. They didn't eat calories; they ate food! And after seeing the same thing time and time again whilst travelling around the world, I started getting the message; I replaced my blind religious mathematical approach with reality and took notice of the few awakened instincts that started guiding me to the next step in my training and nutrition philosophy.

Since then, I have learnt what food gives me energy, strength, and size and what food makes me bloated, sluggish, and slow. I have recognised the difference between the food that helps me to burn body fat vs. food that makes me fat. I have learnt when to stop eating, how many meals per day give me the best results, what foods relieve stress, and what foods make me nervous and edgy. After implementing the changes, I started improving dramatically, winning competitions, controlling my size and body-fat levels with amazing precision and without the excessive effort and struggles of the past. I became more optimistic, more motivated, more self-confident and much happier once I also started feeling, rather than just thinking how to train and eat properly. After experiencing all these great changes in myself, I started helping others using the same principles and approach, and since then I have achieved amazing results with thousands of clients from all around the globe.

The major reason for the total failure of the dry mathematical approach lays in the misunderstanding of human nature and physiology — that very complex, dynamic and ever-changing, almost unpredictable life machinery. When we say that metabolism is the sum of all chemical processes which occur in the body, we actually say very little; metabolism means much more than that! Let's just start with breathing, blood oxygenation, oxygen distribution, CO_2 removal, production of vitamin D in the skin, production of red and white blood cells, immunity, nerve impulses, liver function and enzyme production, and we just begin to see the story of metabolism going on and on and on... For every single process in the body, chemical and mechanical, energy is needed, energy that is measured in calories. Now, how accurate or possible is it to be able predict the daily expenditure of calories needed just for basic metabolic needs (maintaining life)? How accurate can anyone be in predicting something so dynamic and so unpredictable? And at the end of the day, why do this? The reason can only be to satisfy a mathematical mind that likes to organize life into numbers, in order to control it and manipulate it.

Experts always talk about daily caloric needs by using the same phrases: "average person", "needs around 2 000 calories", "estimated", "you may expect" and many others phrases that have been used as core terminology in building the hypothetical theories relating to caloric consumption. Knowing about the energy values of food and its caloric density is very important for identifying foods that can make us fatter more easily or foods that will satisfy us, yet contain far fewer calories. But all calories are not the same; calories from sugar are not the same as calories from protein or essential fats. Knowing the difference between empty calories and calories with real nutritional value is crucial in order to correctly assess the quality of food that we eat daily. Extra information can never hurt anyone, but when we try to manipulate certain issues with the wrong intellectual tools, the result in terms of human nutrition can be very costly.

An individual's metabolism changes all the time, it has no constant value. If we try to evaluate daily energetic output, for example, we cannot assume that the result for one day will be applicable on an everyday basis. Depending on many different circumstances, our metabolism will require more or fewer calories from one day to the next. Chemical processes within the body change constantly with different dynamics. To look at some of the very sensitive changes that occur constantly throughout every 24-hour period, let's start with the hormonal system. The amount and type of hormones released after every meal we eat depends on the type of food we eat, our emotional state, our catabolic or anabolic prevalence at a particular time of the day, as well as many other factors. Our liver functions depend on the type of food we eat, stress levels on a daily basis, medication (if taken), amount of alcohol and saturated fat that we consume daily, hormonal balance, infections, inflammation, etc. Our digestive activities depend on the amount, type and state of food that we eat (raw or cooked), enzyme production, liver health, peristaltic patterns, physical activities, hormonal balance, etc. These are just a few of the ever-changing vital functions that occur constantly throughout our lives. The complexity and dynamics of this marvellous synergy maintaining life suggests strongly that simply counting calories and playing mind games with food will take us nowhere.

Food has to be understood differently, not just as a simple sum of its components and energetic variables which can be measured in energy units known as calories. Calorie games are the most simplistic attempt to understand the nature of food in order to benefit our health. But they simply don't work. Instead, food has to be taken as it has been given to us, to sustain and support life. We eat to live; we don't live to eat! Our instincts should be driving us into the right selection and amount of food that we need in order to live healthily, not to satisfy artificial or induced cravings. The scientific knowledge that we have accumulated over the centuries should help us to get back to ourselves and awaken all our life forces in order to smell, feel, taste and see the premier source of health — food.

The bottom line

- The caloric valuation of food is important in order to understand the amount of energy present in different foods. Foods that contain high amounts of calories, like all processed foods, should be eaten in smaller amounts whilst foods that contains fewer calories, such as fruit and vegetables, fish and lean meats should be eaten in greater amounts.
- The confusion that often stems from the caloric calculation of food starts when all calories are identified as equal. All calories are definitely not the same. Although 4 calories from sugar may equal 4 calories from protein on paper, their destiny and effect on the human body is totally different.

Fasting

Fasting has been part of human life for thousands of years. Whilst the absence of food for relatively short periods of time, i.e. 1 – 7 days, due to varying success in hunting and gathering has been regarded as normal for most of our evolution, the absence of food has been understood as a punishment in modern times — something very bad for our health and even sometimes disastrous. For most of our history, food wasn't available everywhere, at any time and in any desired amount. Despite the beliefs of some nutritionists — especially the ones who attempt to prove that we evolved mainly around fruits and vegetables — the Garden of Eden scenario is very unlikely. In most parts of the world, vegetables and fruits are still, as they have always been, only a seasonal opportunity. Animal food is the only food that is and was available then and now at all times. Hunting animals successfully during times when fruits and vegetables weren't available (especially during the ice ages) didn't guarantee food on a daily basis. It simply meant that if the animal or fish wasn't caught then, there wouldn't be any food for the day!

Periods of fasting were thus a normal part of life, sometimes shorter, sometimes longer in duration, but the absence of food has been a part of the human experience more often than the continued abundance of food. The questions that we can ask today are: did this absence of food do more good or harm for our ancestors, and can we actually benefit from the occasional absence of food or from fasting? Is there anything good that can come out of infrequent, occasional fasting, or will the occasional absence of food create a risk to our health?

If you take a closer look at the world's largest religions, you will notice that every one of them advocates fasting in one form or another. They can be either fasting from sunrise to sunset every day for a month in Islam, or the absence of certain foods on some days of the year in Christianity, for example. Although religions have introduced regular fasting more for the purposes of mental and spiritual purification, at least formally, the origins of fasting are really physiological.

The digestion of food is not an easy process for the body. Digestion requires a lot of energy and effort, which can result in weakened immunity. The ability of the body to protect itself from infections and diseases is what is meant by immunity, and it requires a lot of energy. If you spend most of your energy dealing with digestive system emergencies, like for example eating the wrong combination of food, there will be less energy left for your immune system. Eating a lot of saturated and hydrogenated fats and refined starches and sugars will do the same thing — it will take lots of energy for digesting the same food and then detoxifying from it. So guess what our reality as far as eating food is today? Most of us eat the wrong food in the wrong combinations, which sucks most of our energy out, leaving a weakened immune system. Are you one of those people who think that it is normal to have the flu twice a year? No, it's not normal! The wrong diet is the most important reason for people getting common infections and suffering from chronic disease like diabetes, cardiovascular diseases and others. Lowering immunity by shifting most of the life energy into digestion is unfortunately the most common situation for the majority of people today.

During illness, when most of the body's energy is directed towards the immune system, wasting energy on digestion (and most likely the wrong food and wrong combination of food) would be a poor choice for the body. So what does the body do in these situations? It suppresses appetite and concentrates on eliminating the problem. This is exactly when the reasons for fasting come into play. Even without any health problems, the human body benefits from occasional fasting. As long as fasting is understood and undertaken carefully and deliberately for health reasons, great benefits can be expected.

Although the basic idea of fasting means the forced (but voluntary) absence of food for a certain period of time, there are still variations of reducing only certain types of food for certain periods of time in order to come close to the benefits of total fasting. For example, when you eliminate some basic types of food from your diet for a day or few days, like starches and protein food, you will still benefit from a reduction of overall stress to the digestive system. Eating only different vegetables for 2 - 3 days will help a lot to rest the digestive system. It will also rest the liver and pancreas, which are major enzyme producers, as well as eliminate toxins, allow more energy for the immune system, etc.

A constant intake of simple sugars, saturated fats, starches and even protein in high amounts, puts a huge stress on the digestive and other systems without giving them a break. The build-up of the toxic by-products of digestion, toxified tissues (cells) and the extra body fat that usually accompany the over-eating of wrong foods are all consequences of a permanent bombardment of the wrong ingredients. When the major food groups that mainly contribute to toxic build-up get eliminated from the diet even for a day or so, the body has an opportunity to recover itself and eliminate undigested remains from the digestive tract and some of the intoxicated cells and body fat, whilst producing more of the hormones that rejuvenate the body and also burn extra body fat (for example, growth hormone).

When people understand the importance of fasting and decide to start experimenting with it, it's very important to begin with caution and patience. This is the major reason to first start a fasting experience with relatively gentle forms of fasting in order to prepare the body for more extreme total fasting later on. Total fasting means the absence of all foods for a period of time (with the exception of water) and represents the most intense detoxification process, one undertaken only by natural methods of food elimination, not with the help of medications. There are a few different stages of fasting that have to be understood and considered before you begin, however. One should always start with a less drastic type of fasting and slowly adapt and get ready for more intense fasting.

After many years of improper eating and overeating on a daily basis, your body will struggle with, rather than benefit from, immediate total fasting. This is the reason why you should start your first fasting experience with a diet that consists only of fruits for one day. A fruit-only diet for one or two days will eliminate the build-up of toxins in the body and force the body to rely on other energy sources like body fat and unneeded tissues (cells) in the body. Fruits are very easy to digest, and also provide lots of fibre and natural detoxifiers like antioxidants without heavily engaging the digestive system. Whilst on the fruit diet, your body will satisfy its need for essential amino acids for vital organs from skeletal muscle tissues. The fruit days may be substituted with fruit juice days. Some people prefer to drink fruit rather than eat it. I still believe that eating fruit is a much better option than drinking it, simply because while you chew fruit your digestive juices are secreted even before the fruit enters the stomach. Our teeth, gums and jaws are designed for chewing and they will perform best and last longer if we use them to their full capacity. When you squeeze or press fruit to make juice (5 - 6 apples are needed to make a single glass of apple juice) you skip over the natural chewing process and just swallow the juice. The truth is that you will benefit more from the parts of the fruit that are separated from the juice and end up in your garbage bin! This is why I always advise and prefer eating fruits rather than drinking only juice. Although marketing fruit juices has greatly helped juicer manufacturers, it hasn't helped inform the general public about the reality of digesting and absorbing the food with maximum results and without the risk of unhealthy intestinal irritation.

Once you gain some experience in fasting only on fruit for a day or a few days, and repeat it a few times over a period of 3 - 4 months, you will be ready to enter the next stage of fasting that consists of eating only vegetables.

Fruits and vegetables are excellent natural detoxifiers, but they have a different impact on the digestive system and the body's biochemistry in general. Both of these are natural foods high in essential minerals, vitamins, enzymes and fibre. Both fruits and vegetables improve the digestion of other foods and are digested without a major impact on the digestive system. Although they can supply different micronutrients and fibre to the body, the major difference between them is in the amount and type of sugars that they contain. Fruits contain more sugars than vegetables and therefore bring more energy and calories into the body. Most fruit contains around 12% sugar, whilst most vegetables contain only around 3%. By switching from fruit fasts to vegetable fasts, you will force your body to eliminate toxins and by-products to a greater degree. The reason for this lies in the fact that fruit sugar will replace the liver glycogen, and the body will be reluctant to dip into the body fat for its energy needs as it will do in a situation when carbohydrates are not around.

Fruit and vegetables are both easily digested by the body, so there is no burden to the digestive system from them, and no particular benefit in drinking juices instead of eating fruits and vegetables, apart from convenience.

Fasting only on vegetable juices is another option, and there are people who have achieved great results with vegetable juice fasts. For the same reasons mentioned above, I would still prefer to eat vegetables rather than to drink them; the benefits of eating food rather than "drinking" it are naturally obvious.

Fruit and vegetables are also very rich in fibre and water, as well as in micronutrients like minerals and vitamins. All of these components are extremely good toxin eliminators for the body. When you stop eating protein and starchy food for a day or more, the purifying effect of the fruit and vegetables will increase.

After trying the above steps you may ask why you would need to do anything more, such as total fasting, in order to cleanse the body? Well, fasting only on water for a day or more (up to 7 days) is the most intense type of fasting possible and will take you from cleaning your digestive system of fermented carbohydrates and putrefied protein particles and other by-products of digestion that may have been stuck in the intestines, to cellular cleansing by faster elimination of dead cells, degenerated cells and even cancer cells. Loss of body fat is also accelerated while on a total fast rather than on a fast that permits fruit and vegetables.

Fasting only on water is the most drastic type of fasting and requires experience. In cases of prolonged fasting without any food, the person who is on the fast may require medical supervision. A water-only fast should start first with a one day fast, then be repeated in a few weeks, progressing to 2 or 3 days in duration. For a longer duration total fast, one needs to have previous experience with some type of fasting. Working slowly, gradually build up your total fasting ability over a period of a few months if you are planning to fast for longer than three days.

The typical side-effects experienced during a total fast are low energy levels, light-headedness, nausea and irritability. These symptoms usually disappear after 2 - 3 days when the body starts running on its own body fat and ketones as a main source of fuel. The first visible result of short fasting (2 - 3 days) is weight loss. Some 3 - 6 pounds may be lost in the first 2 - 3 days of fasting. That weight loss derives mainly from stuck, undigested food in the digestive tract, extra retained water, lean muscle tissue and some body fat. Weight lost during these kinds of fasts should not be considered as fat loss only! Losing only body fat is a very complicated process and requires the perfect combination of effective exercises and a muscle-preserving, fat-burning diet.

Apart from the physical cleansing of removing undigested food particles from the digestive system, your body will also benefit from a cleansing at the cellular level, a rested digestive system and elimination of different accumulated acids when subjected to a total fast. Alkaline foods such as vegetables and fruits will lower the acidity in the body, while natural mineral water with a pH balance of 7 will also help to maintain the body's optimum pH level.

It's important to remember that breaking a fast should be done gradually. This means that once you have decided to stop fasting you should only reintroduce food slowly. Your first meal after a total fast should just be a piece of fruit, the second some light yoghurt, and the third meal can consist of some protein source like chicken with vegetables. The following day you can continue to eat as before, healthily and regularly.

The bottom line

- Fasting (or more precisely involuntary hunger) has been a natural experience for humans for most of our evolution.
- Though it may not have been deliberate, hunger is a natural state around which we have adapted for hundreds of thousands of years.
- For millennia we have been hunters and gatherers and food was never guaranteed on a daily basis.
- Nowadays we have access to all kinds of food at any time and that is not doing us good. Occasional fasting can help us become even healthier.
- Fasting is the elimination of all food or some types of food for a certain period of time.
- There are different levels of fasting, total fasting being the most drastic type, where all food is eliminated and only water is allowed for a certain period of time.
- Fasting can help us detoxify and strengthen immunity, by eliminating undigested food particles from the digestive system, losing extra water and body fat and also by detoxifying the body at a cellular level.
- Fasting should be introduced slowly and in stages.

Breaking the Myths

There are a lot of myths surrounding the complex issue of nutrition that help to worsen human health in general. Chronic diseases, the biggest killer of humans, have been in constant increase since the discovery of agriculture and we now know that they are directly related to the food that we eat. Although other factors like stress, inactivity and poor lifestyle in general cannot be discounted, food is still the single most powerful factor when it comes to human health. In this chapter I will try to break some of the most common nutritional myths that are diverting our focus and preventing our full understanding of healthy eating.

Myth number 1 - The food pyramid

In the "officially" recognized food pyramid that has been advocated by the medical community, the bottom of the pyramid is made up of some 70% carbohydrates. The next layer in the middle,constituting 20% of the pyramid, is dedicated to fat, and the last level of the pyramid - only 10% - is dedicated to protein. This food pyramid has been used as a starting point for creating supposedly healthy diets in recent times. These "healthy" diets have been made up mainly of carbohydrates (around 70%) with some fat and very little protein. In order to adhere to this model and maintain 70% of the daily diet from carbohydrates, the main food choice has to be the complex carbohydrates found in grains, since they are highly concentrated and the only ones that would be possible to eat to maintain such a proportion of nutrients. It is impossible to eat natural sources of carbohydrates like fruits and vegetables to the point where they comprise 70% of our daily caloric intake!

Because this food pyramid guided diet is mainly made from easily digestible energy food, the only way to control someone's normal bodyweight would be to restrict the number of calories eaten daily. As we all know though, low-calorie diets do not work, simply because of the heavy deprivation of calories on a daily basis and the limited amount of protein that is essential for tissue growth and repair. Depriving the body of the most essential macronutrient, protein, will cause food cravings that will spoil every attempt to succeed with a low-calorie diet. Low caloric intake, the only option for a mostly carbohydrate-based diet will never work over the long term. Exposed to a low-calorie diet for an extended period of time, the body will move into starvation mode, slowing down its metabolism and preserving fat tissue at the expense of muscle tissue. The weight loss that occurs from such a diet comes mainly from muscle tissue rather than body fat. Needless to say, this is the worst scenario for every dieter. In order to retrieve the muscle tissue necessary for a healthy metabolism and all around daily activities, the body will constantly trigger the hunger mechanism by craving calories (protein) and eventually hunger will win. This is the all-too-familiar outcome for most of the dieters that have attempted to lose weight on a high-carbohydrate, low-calorie diet. What almost always results at the end of such a diet is binge overeating for days, even weeks, and all the lost weight will come back along with a few new pounds of extra fat.

The major cause of this unwanted eating pattern lays in the acceptance of the incorrectly structured food pyramid as a fundamental dietary principle. However, gaining a few pounds of extra body fat, although not healthy, is not the worst consequence that will come from this suggested high carbohydrate diet. The vicious insulin cycle will create a constant need for carbohydrates, which will then create a higher demand for insulin. So, the constant need for carbohydrates created by low blood sugar level due to high insulin presence and overproduction of insulin due to high presence of carbohydrates is the best recipe for low insulin sensitivity, glucose intolerance and diabetes.

Myth number 2 - Food groups

It has often been said that no single food group should be avoided in any type of diet. I totally agree with this as long as the food groups are selected from a natural menu rather than from the menu made by profit making companies and advocates of political correctness in nutrition. I agree that political correctness is an important factor that has to be taken into consideration, but I can't ignore the message that has been delivered by the actual reality of the situation. This message is that the health of the nation is constantly deteriorating due to the wrong dietary advice.

The only food groups that we have to take into consideration in order to deliver a safe dietary experience are natural foods like meat, fish, fruits and vegetables. What I call natural foods are the foods that can be eaten in the form and shape as nature provides them to us, without any processing. Natural foods can be eaten raw, in a fresh state. Even meat and fish can be eaten raw, and in this state they can deliver all the goodness of the micro and macronutrients in a non-spoiled state. Cooking, boiling, baking and any other way of exposing food to high temperatures involves processing the food. Processing food in this manner simply deactivates enzymes, vitamins and most of the minerals while greatly lowering the absorption level of proteins. These are the foods known to the human species for millions of years and human physiology has developed successfully around only these types of foods until now. Any other edibles introduced into our diet in recent history, like grains and milk products, have caused us health problems, chronic disease being the deadliest. Grains cannot be eaten raw — they have to be heavily processed before delivered to your plate, ready to eat. Just think for a second about bread, pasta and rice! The art of processing them seems never ending and the food becomes dead many times before you eat it.

The idea of implementing all food groups together actually started in order to defend grains and dairy products, granting them a dominant presence in our daily diet. By identifying them as legitimate food groups, their promoters managed to implement them successfully into the very misleading food pyramid that we have been indoctrinated into believing as a new eleventh commandment! This has thus become a "Holy Grail" with no comments wanted or permitted!

Myth number 3 - Carbohydrates are the body's most preferable source of energy

For some unjustified reasons, carbohydrates have become the primary choice for energy food. Foods rich in carbohydrates, like grains, have become staple foods simply because they are easy to produce and are packed with the most calories. Are you still wondering why meat and fish are much more expensive than bread and pasta? Protein-rich food is much more difficult to produce, yet interestingly enough, protein-rich food does not contain any carbohydrates.

It seems like the good old saying has been proven right again: quality doesn't come cheap.

When it comes to energy sources for the body, there are three main sources of macronutrients that our body can use for energy: protein, fat and carbohydrates. The human body can use them all in order to produce the energy needed for everyday life activities. For most of our history, fat and protein have been the primary sources of energy for humans. For the majority of our evolution carbohydrates have only been available in the form of vegetables or fruit. These foods are not high in carbohydrates — no more than 12% in fruit and around 4% in vegetables — and they are mainly seasonally available in many regions of the world. The only food that has been constantly available for human consumption is meat and in relatively recent history, fish. Being dense in protein and fat but not in carbohydrates, meat and fish have produced abundance in calories and provided all the energy needed to survive and continue the species without passing chronic diseases to successive generations. The major reason for that "safe" energy delivered from fat and protein is that neither fat nor protein require high amounts of insulin in order to be delivered to the other tissues in the form of fatty or amino acids. Carbohydrates were never the primary source of energy for humans. It was always fat and protein, followed by carbohydrates from fruit and vegetables. This is why we have never adapted to high-carbohydrate diets or developed the ability to safely digest and absorb them in high quantities.

Why are they then marketed as the preferable source of energy? The truth is that carbohydrates are the most easily digestible macronutrient. It takes much less effort and energy to digest carbohydrates than protein and it takes much less energy for the body to make energy from dietary carbohydrates then from dietary fat or stored body fat. But being the easiest to digest, carbohydrates also provide too much quick energy to the blood causing the hormonal imbalance of insulin and glucagon and thus shouldn't be considered the most "desirable" source of energy. Fat and protein never cause a huge surge of blood sugar like carbohydrates do. That sudden and huge increase of blood sugar has been the major cause of our health deterioration in the form of chronic diseases. Something that is easy to digest should not be confused with being "preferable" as a source of energy. It is obvious that wherever carbohydrates prevail over protein and natural fats (in any corner of the world), health problems related to obesity and hyper production of insulin have spread quickly.

Myth number 4 - Eating 6 - 7 smaller meals is better than eating 3 - 4 larger meals

For decades, nutritionists and fitness experts kept repeating the same song that eating several smaller meals on a daily basis is better than eating a few "larger" meals. They have never explained properly why we need to eat so many meals per day in order to keep lean and healthy and why those meals have to be small. The whole concept of eating numerous smaller meals has been built on the idea that the main food component in our diet has to be carbohydrates! For some reason, that premise has been accepted as the Holy Grail and everything had to be built around it. If you consume carbohydrates as 60 - 70% of your diet and you try to build a healthy eating plan around that fundamental premise, you will have to keep your sugar level constant and satisfy the viscous insulin demand throughout the day. In order to avoid getting fat, you will have to keep your glycemic load small and constantly fight the sensation of hunger that will

inevitably occur every 2 - 3 hours on a diet overly rich in carbohydrates. You will simply have to eat more often throughout the day.
So, what will you eat? Small meals every 2 - 3 hours that will provide you with constant energy and at the same time keep you lean?
Is this possible? Yes it is, but it will not last long, simply because
constantly eating small meals will soon turn into constantly eating
much bigger meals (as everyone who has tried this knows very well)!

So, imagine for a minute what would happen if you based your
diet around natural foods (foods that can be eaten without processing). If your diet is created around vegetables, fruits and meats, your
energy providing services will take a completely different turn. In
this scenario, your energy will have to come mainly from dietary
fat or stored body fat. The amount of energy that is available from
body fat is simply unlimited compared to the energy that is available
from dietary carbohydrates. Your body fat stores that are specially
designed to provide you with energy will never fail you. Once your
body turns to the body fat as a major source of energy, your blood
sugar level will stabilise, your cravings will disappear and you will
not experience hunger so often during the day. You will probably
do well with only 3 - 4 reasonably good size meals, meals that may
be large in size, but not that high in caloric value! Meals made from
meat (fish or chicken, etc.) and lots of vegetables are substantial due
to their high water and fibre content, but are not that big in terms of
the caloric load that they provide. These types of meals will satisfy
your hunger for longer and will not cause cravings due to the lack of
protein or other essential nutrients.

What will force you to eat more meals per day is the constant insulin
production that lowers your blood sugar levels and creates hunger
that can only be satisfied with yet another meal. Whether you eat 5,

6 or 8 times per day is totally irrelevant, what is relevant is that you will not be in charge of your eating in this scenario. It will be insulin that is in control, the most powerful, yet at the same time potentially deadliest hormone in your body.

So, if you end up eating only 3 to 4 meals made from meat or fish, lots of vegetables in their natural raw state and essential fats, don't feel guilty. You have just followed the natural way of eating, using hunger to time your meals and supplying your body with all essential amino and fatty acids. If you feel that you want something to eat in between your main meals, fruits and nuts are the best foods to snack on.

Bear in mind that people who are more physically active and have very fast metabolisms, like professional athletes, may eat one or two meals more during the day due to their different metabolic demands. They cannot be taken as typical examples though and the general public should not follow their eating patterns.

The choice of food that you eat during the day will decide every-thing; you will either end up eating as many as 8 - 9 small carbohy-drate-based meals per day, or you will be very happy and energetic with 3 - 4 or even 5 protein and vegetable-based meals per day.

Myth number 5 - You need carbohydrates in order to keep your energy level up during the day

This myth comes out of misunderstanding the source and supply of glucose, the main energy form available for absorption by the human body. If glucose was only available from dietary carbohydrates, the story of energy would be very short and easy to understand. But, the human body has developed many ways of sourcing blood sugar (glucose) from either carbohydrates, fats and/or proteins.

During our evolution, different food sources were available to humans, with meat being the most reliable and consistent food available throughout the year. Human physiology has developed around the most abundant foods, like meat, vegetables, nuts and fruit. Adapting to their living environment, humans have developed physiological responses to the food that has been available for most of the time throughout the year. Protein and fat were there at all times, while vegetables and fruit were only available depending on the time of the year and part of the world (in some parts of the world they were not available at all). Energy levels were kept up mainly by producing glucose from dietary fat and protein (and also from stored energy in the form of glycogen and body fat). Fruits and vegetables were always welcomed, but not the most reliable and energy efficient foods (fruits contain no more than 12% sugar and vegetables no more than 4% sugar). The most valued foods for humans, regarding their energy potential (caloric value) were meat, fish and nuts, all high in fat and protein and therefore high in energy that doesn't require a high production of the troublesome insulin hormone.

Understanding that energy directly depends on blood sugar levels will help you to create the perfect daily diet without causing harm to yourself. Blood sugar (glucose) can be produced from carbohydrates, fats or proteins. Every macronutrient can be turned into blood sugar. While fat and protein don't create a surge of insulin to control glucose, carbohydrates do and have to be controlled. The best sources of carbohydrates are thus fruits and vegetables, simply because they don't contain high amounts of carbohydrates and yet are rich in fibre which further helps to control insulin production. Fruit mainly contains fructose, a type of sugar that doesn't need insulin in order to be metabolised. Eating foods from the natural menu (meats, fish, vegetables, nuts and fruit) is simply a win-win situation.

Eating processed foods like sugar, pasta, bread, rice and different sources of cereals, will provide too much blood sugar too quickly, therefore requiring too much insulin to counter the elevated glucose. Insulin produced in high amounts will do more harm than good to you, creating the potential for developing many different types of chronic diseases and storing the extra sugar in the form of body fat. Eating refined carbohydrates is simply a lose-lose situation.

Myth number 6 - Weight loss

The "weight loss" phenomenon is another getaway for the proponents of diets made from refined foods, mainly carbohydrates. Every one of us is familiar with the terminology of weight loss. But weight loss is a totally fabricated terminology. Weight loss really means nothing, nothing at all! Who ever wanted to lose weight? All that any one of us ever wanted to lose was fat around the knees, thighs, hips and buttocks; fat that likes to remain forever around our waistlines, around our chest and arms and on our necks and faces. What else would anyone want to lose? Body weight? Absolute nonsense. You don't see your body weight in the mirror, all that you see and want to lose is that dead body fat that hangs in the wrong places and gives you that funny shape.

So why were we all hypnotised into believing that it is body weight rather than body fat that should be regulated or lost in order to achieve a healthy or fantastic looking body? The reason why lays in the foundation of the official understanding of nutrition and healthy eating. With the current view of healthy eating, food that is seen as being healthy and diets that are seen as effective for fat loss will never help you to lose fat! The food that is offered and manipulated into the most unnatural diets will, in the best-case scenario, offer you some weight loss, but never from fat loss only!

So, you might ask, what is wrong with weight loss? Well, everything is wrong with weight loss, from my point of view. Weight loss is one thing, but fat loss is something totally different. When you lose weight you never know what kind of body material you have actually lost. In most cases, weight loss is mainly achieved due to loss of water, muscle tissue and only a little body fat. This is the reason why many people end up losing 10 - 15 pounds of body weight, but still retain a lot of fat tissue around their legs, or waistline! You may end up with that stringy look, but your body will not be tight and vibrant, especially in the most critical areas like legs, buttocks and waistline.

When I talk about fat loss I'm not concerned with weight loss at all! A diet based on natural foods will provide you with the essential macro and micronutrients that will stimulate your metabolism to preserve lean body tissues and use body fat as the main source of energy. The final product of this approach will be a very tight and lean body, full of energy and maintaining a vibrant healthy look. In combination with an effective exercise program, your extra body fat (in case you have any) will simply disappear without any big fuss, and what is most important, you will preserve your new look and great health as long as you follow a healthy lifestyle. It's fat loss that matters, not weight loss!

Myth number 7 - If you want to lose weight you have to eat carbohydrates and cut the fat out of your diet

This myth is based on the simple mathematics of counting calories. Because carbohydrates contain only 4 calories per gram while fat contains 9 calories per gram, it seems that if you eat carbohydrates instead of fat you will reduce your overall amount of calorie consumption. This myth also assumes that all fats are the same, simply because their energy values are expressed in calories. Yes, it is true that all fats have the same caloric value (they all contain 9 calories per gram), but while they all have the same energy potential, they are far from being the same. There are fats which are essential for the human body and there are fats which are not. Simply said, there are good fats and bad fats.

If counting calories was the most important skill in the fight against extra body weight in the form of fat, everyone would be lean! But in reality, as we all know, the actual situation is very different. The hysteria against fat intake has spread around the developed world and has resulted in hundreds, if not thousands of different products that are very low in fat or even fat-free! At the same time, the so-called "healthy" low-fat products happen to be very high in carbohydrates. Among the worst examples of these are breakfast and other cereals, most of them containing over 70% carbohydrates. Next in line are a whole army of products that follow like fat-free biscuits, fat-free chocolates, fat-free muffins, fat-free ice cream, fat-free bread, fat-free salad dressings, fat-free chocolate drinks, fat-free fruit yoghurts and many more similar products that are packed with carbohydrates and at the same time carry a huge amount of calories. And although we are now surrounded as never before with hundreds of "healthy" fat-free products, we are still getting fatter than we ever have! The paradox is that we were much leaner as a nation back when there were no fat-free products and when people ate more fat than we eat nowadays!

Obviously, the reason for weight (fat) gain, especially in the last 20 years in the developed world, is the dramatically increased consumption of carbohydrates. Even if lower in calories per single gram than fat, carbohydrates are eaten in huge amounts, as advised by nutrition authorities, contributing to the high energy intake and detrimental hormonal imbalancing of the body. By overproducing insulin and lowering the production of glucagons, fat accumulation is unavoidable. The fine-tuning of insulin and glucagons in the optimal, beneficial proportion for everyone is only possible if a natural type of diet is followed — a diet rich in meat, fish, vegetables and fruit. Only these foods will allow the body to use carbohydrates and fats as its main sources of energy and operate at its optimal efficiency without producing dangerous levels of insulin.

While fats are essential for human health, carbohydrates are not! Good fats, like the ones found in ocean fish, grass-fed animals, nuts and vegetables are necessary for healthy living. These fats have been present in our daily diets since we first walked the earth. Fat is also essential for the absorption of crucial vitamins like vitamins E, A, D and K. Without fat present in the daily diet we would suffer from deficiencies of the fat-soluble vitamins which are essential for immunity, calcium absorption and other vital functions in the body. Fat that has been manufactured in order to maintain the longer shelf life of modern commercial products (hydrogenated fats) are not healthy for us and have to be avoided. These fats are usually present in most of the processed foods we find today.

Even fats found in meat should not be demonised. In naturally raised animals, the amount of fat is not as high as in animals that are commercially raised. If you have no other option but to buy meat that is not naturally raised, try to buy lean beef or pork cuts, chicken, turkey breasts or liver — all low in fat. Grass-fed livestock is naturally leaner and the types of fat in their meat are also different than in animals that are raised faster with processed foods. Bison, venison, rabbit, ostrich and similar wild meats grown naturally are low in saturated fat but at the same time higher in essential fats than farmed livestock. Choose ocean wild fish over farmed fish as the overall amount of fat in them is lower while the amount of essential fats is higher.

Carbohydrates should be consumed through natural foods like vegetables and fruit. The amount and type of carbohydrates that come from such foods is ideal for human health. They will never require high amounts of insulin and by providing high amounts of fibre, they will help digestion, assimilation and elimination of by-products.

As this myth has suggested, a high carbohydrate intake mainly from grains and a very low amount of dietary fat in order to attempt to lose excess body fat will simply cause the opposite to happen. As we all know, a diet based on low-fat products and high carbohydrate intake has created levels of obesity that have never been seen before. Many cases of malnutrition, which is a lack of essential vitamins in the body, are also related to low-fat, high carbohydrate diets. High carbohydrate diets also tend to be very low in protein and consequently in the essential amino acids necessary for tissue repair and growth. And once again, while there are essential amino acids and fatty acids, there are no essential carbohydrates. This means that we have no physiological needs for carbohydrates like we do for proteins and fat!

Myth number 8 - Complex carbohydrates are better than simple sugars

When carbohydrates become the main macronutrient in the diet, problems will occur. An increase in body fat is the first sign of the impact of carbohydrates on one's diet. In high-carbohydrate diets, protein is usually the main macronutrient to suffer since it's heavily neglected in favour of carbohydrates. A low protein intake results in loss of muscle tissue since muscles have to be used as a source of amino acids necessary for the repair and maintenance of internal organs like the heart, lung, liver and others. As we know, in regions of the world where people's survival depends on foods high in carbohydrates such as grains and grain products, protein and essential micronutrient malnutrition is a common problem. I have experienced the same problem with numerous clients who, for cultural or religious reasons, followed diets based mainly on carbohydrates. A high level of body fat and very weak muscular development always follows diets high in carbohydrates and low in high quality animal protein.

In light of so many negative consequences for human health from carbohydrate-heavy diets, the only escape route for carbohydrate proponents is to find something good about them. The main attempt has been to split carbohydrates into good and bad kinds — thus we have ended up with the "great" health benefits of complex carbohydrates and "bad" health consequences of simple carbohydrates. We have finally gotten a bad boys vs. good boys scenario! According to the advocates of high-carbohydrate diets, all we have to worry about are simple sugars: mainly table sugar, sucrose, and everything containing them. As long as we stay away from them and stick to complex sugars like the ones found in grains, potatoes and their products (porridge, cereals, brown bread, starch, etc.) we will be alright.

The idea of calorie-controlled diets has become a cornerstone of recent nutrition theory thanks to this rationalization. But having understood that a high-carbohydrate diet makes people fat without exception, the advocates of this diet have turned their efforts to a diet that will eliminate the devastating effects of the phenomenon of fat accumulation. By trying their best in constructing something that the human race never attempted before (a calorie-restricted diet), the engineers of this new approach had to keep the dominance of carbohydrates in the diet while still offering a calorie restriction solution. In this scenario, complex carbohydrates have come out ahead, while the suggested amount of daily protein ended up being very low. In a calorie-restricted diet, where carbohydrates dominate, there is simply no room for protein or fat.

Complex carbohydrates have been offered as a better solution in calorie-restricted diets rather than simple carbohydrates like sugar. Because they are made of more complex molecules that have to first be broken down into glucose, complex carbohydrates take longer to be digested and induce less insulin production than simple carbohydrates. Unlike simple carbohydrates that enter the blood very quickly and require a high amount of insulin, complex carbohydrates enter the blood more slowly due to their more complex molecular structure, and need less insulin for their transport to either glycogen or fat stores around the body. Everything would be fine if the story of complex carbohydrates ended at this point. If there were nothing else but glycemic index, the whole complex carbohydrates affair would be simple. But, is it?

Apart from glycemic index, there is also something called glycemic load, the measure that matters more to our health than glycemic index alone. Glycemic load represents the TOTAL amount of carbohydrates eaten daily multiplied by their glycemic index. The final sum gives a much better picture of one's daily intake of food (carbohydrates) than just glycemic index by itself. For example, if you ate 300 grams of oats with an average glycemic index of 45, the glycemic index would be 300 x 45 = 13 500. If, on the other hand, you ate 100 grams of white rice with a glycemic index of 70, the total would be 100 x 70 = 7 000. In the second case your glycemic load will be smaller than in the first case – 7 000 versus 13 500. To process the carbohydrates you would without doubt need to produce insulin in sufficient amounts. With the higher glycemic load the daily amount of carbohydrates will require more insulin in total, even though there was a lower glycemic index!

Although glycemic index will help you to understand the release speed of particular carbohydrates in the blood (where slow-releasing carbohydrates are preferred over fast-releasing carbohydrates) the overall amount of carbohydrates eaten on a daily basis still represents the most important factor in everyone's diet.

Carbohydrates once again should only be eaten in the required amounts. In the majority of cases, people overeat carbohydrates regardless of their glycemic index, making the glycemic load too high. The necessary amount of carbohydrates for most of us can easily be satisfied by eating enough fruits and vegetables each day. They will not only provide the "necessary" amount of carbohydrates (which is relatively low compared to our modern understanding of healthy eating), but also the right amounts of minerals and vitamins which are necessary for the digestion and absorption of carbohydrates in the first place. The high level of fibre in fruit and vegetables will also slow down their absorption and therefore demand lower insulin production when eaten.

So, the myth that complex carbohydrates are better than simple carbohydrates is only partially true and often misleading. By branding them better and safe, they have been granted a dominant and primary role in the everyday diets of a majority of people. I still encounter on a daily basis, the confusion people have who follow an apparently "healthy" diet full of complex carbohydrates and low in protein and fat but still have weight problems!

Complex carbohydrates and simple carbohydrates are both carbohydrates regardless. They are made of the same molecules of carbon and hydrogen, the only difference being the length of the chain of carbon molecules in each particular carbohydrate. Complex ones have longer molecular carbon chains and therefore require a longer time to be broken down into simple sugars. OVEREATING complex carbohydrates results in grave consequences — so, why do we OVEREAT complex carbohydrates? This million-dollar question has been troubling the medical authorities for decades. There should be no sympathy for either simple or complex carbohydrates. Once you favour any of them you will be giving a green light to unlimited consumption of either one.

In my long career, I have never known anyone to eat complex or simple carbohydrates in moderation, or even in a best-case scenario, in limited amounts. Carbohydrates, whether complex or simple, at the end of the day require insulin as the only carrier and storage hormone that has to deliver them to the body's cells (muscles, liver and fat cells). Any more of any type of carbohydrate consumption will create a high amount of insulin, causing the chain of negative side effects from over production of the most powerful and also most potentially damaging hormone in the human body.

The dominance of complex carbohydrates in modern diets around the world is obvious. Grains in the form of bread, cereals, rice and other grain products are the dominant components in modern diets. People are fooling themselves believing that breakfasts made of cereals and lunches made of brown bread are the best dietary choices. The results of this type of eating shown in the health statistics of today from around the world speak louder than any critics. We are simply becoming worse off by making complex carbohydrates such a predominant component in our daily diets.

Myth number 9 - Too much protein will make you fat

We have all heard that people in western societies eat more protein than they need, and that over-consumption of protein is one of the major causes of weight gain and deteriorating health. For the reasons I have already described, protein cannot be implemented in high-carbohydrate diets except in very small amounts. From the advocates of high-carbohydrate diets, we have ended up with the advice that a man weighing 90 kilograms has to eat a maximum of 90 grams of protein per day or otherwise face negative health consequences. In reality though, this formula means that that someone weighing 90 kilograms should eat no more than 23 grams of protein per meal if he eats 4 times per day, or 16 grams of protein per meal if he eats 5 times per day! Do you have any idea what this really means in actual practice? This micro amount of protein consumption is woefully inadequate for any healthy man weighing 90 kilograms and being reasonably physically active during the day. 16 grams of protein per meal would never satisfy anyone, neither man nor woman, not to mention someone weighing 90 kilograms!

This inadequate amount of suggested protein has been contrived in order to maintain and defend the high complex-carbohydrate diet for some reason. So anything higher than 16 grams of protein per meal would be categorised as too much and would apparently destroy your health, in particular your liver, kidneys and large intestine!

Interestingly enough, all these same internal organs have suffered heavily, mainly from the consequences caused by diabetes, one of the deadliest diseases of our modern (carbohydrate-eating) society. Do I need to remind you that diabetes is caused by the overeating of carbohydrates, not the overeating of protein?

The idea of overeating protein only appeared in human history during modern times when carbohydrates became staple foods. Humans were always struggling to find and eat enough protein. Whenever they would catch it and kill it, they would eat as much as they possibly could, never knowing when the next high-protein meal would arrive. I cannot possibly imagine that they would stop after a few bites of fresh meat in order to avoid protein overeating! The idea of overeating protein was and still is the biggest nonsense in the science of nutrition, if I may say so. We all know very well that it is almost impossible to overeat meat or fish. You can only have so much and you will simply stop after eating 250 or 350 grams of beef or tuna steak (if you can eat that much in the first place). After eating that amount of meat or fish you will feel satisfied, full and no longer crave any type of additional food.

Now imagine eating rice, noodles, bread or ice cream and remind yourself of the amount of those foods that you need to eat in order to give you the satisfaction and feeling of fullness. You will simply keep eating such foods not just to the point where you are satisfied, but to the point when you are physically full and cannot eat any more because it will hurt! You can overeat carbohydrates to the point where your calorie consumption per single meal can reach a few thousand calories! In order to reach 1 000 calories from a single protein meal, it would be simply impossible because you would have to eat 250 grams of protein in a single meal, which would account for 1 500 grams of steak! But eating 250 grams of carbohydrates from bread, or ice cream (which is easily eaten in one go while watching a favourite film on TV), or 250 grams or more of carbohydrates from pasta in one meal is an everyday reality for a majority of people in our society.

The myth that too much protein will make you fat is simply not founded on any empirical evidence. Overeating protein is simply impossible! The only problem that occurs is when you decide that 70% of your diet has to be composed of carbohydrates. Only then, and in that scenario, will you find it necessary to limit protein intake. Only in that scenario does the overeating of protein become a threat, which therefore has to be eliminated. In reality, as all the primarily protein-eating indigenous cultures still prove, the practice of overeating protein is non-existent and even impossible to engage in.

Eating too much protein will make you fat ONLY if you overeat carbohydrates, as at that point any amount of protein added on top of the carbs will increase overall caloric consumption that will make you fat. So, it's not overconsumption of protein that makes you fat, but overconsumption of calories through too many carbohydrates in the first place. If your diet is based on protein and vegetables with some fruit between main meals, you will only be eating ENOUGH protein, never too much. Your overall caloric intake will always be much lower than a diet that is based on complex carbohydrates.

In my own experience, I never eat more than 250 - 300 grams of chicken or fish per single meal combined with vegetables in the same meal. I always end my meal feeling completely satisfied and usually don't feel hungry for the next 3 - 4 hours. I do not experience cravings for any food and always feel very energetic. I eat 4 - 5 times per day, mainly protein-based meals combined with vegetables and I maintain a low body fat level while still training with high intensity 5 - 6 times per week. I have never gained fat on a high-protein diet. Every time that I have introduced some complex carbohydrates into my diet, I would always lose my definition and gain unwanted body fat.

Myth number 10 - Red meat is bad for you

Red meat has been the main source of food for humans throughout our evolution. Although a lot of nutrition authors try to devalue red meat and lower its importance in the human diet to maintain their high carbohydrate bias, red meat has offered incomparable benefits to human physiological and mental development. Throughout evolution, different cultures that thrived mainly on meat have enjoyed good health and an absence of all chronic disease that we simply cannot prevent with our modern diets. Even cultures that still mainly eat meat these days don't suffer from chronic diseases at the level that others eating high-carbohydrate diets do.

Red meat has been eaten by humans throughout our evolution. However, the difference between the meat that we eat today and the meat that was eaten by our ancestors is substantial. Our ancestors ate meat from animals that only ate naturally provided food: grass. Animals fed on grass had much less fat around and inside their muscles and body organs, while furthermore, the fat that they accumulated was of a different amount and nature than that of modern farm-raised animals.

Today we eat much more fat from red meat (farmed cattle) and far more saturated fats than ever before. The reason for this is that farmed animals today are fed with grains and even with meat itself, foods that are not meant for them to eat in the first place! Cows are supposed to eat grass, not grains! This is the reason why the red meat on our plates contains too much fat not only in terms of quantity but also in terms of quality (the wrong type of fat).

The best advice that can be given to anyone wanting to still benefit from the richness of red meat is that their choice should always be "lean" red meat, whether it comes from beef, pork or lamb. Lean cuts of red meat offer more benefits and less fat.

The benefits of lean red meat are vast. Red meat is packed with the highest quality protein: complete protein. Complete protein is the protein that contains all essential amino acids necessary for the growth and repair of all our tissues.

Apart from protein, red meat is full of essential micronutrients that are necessary for human health and development. The minerals iron and zinc are abundant in red meat. The iron in meat is mainly heme iron, the most easily absorbed form of iron for humans. Eating red meat also enhances the absorption of iron from plant food. Beef contains 2.7 mg of iron per 100 grams.

Meat is also rich in the essential mineral zinc that plays an important role in the formation of over a hundred different enzymes involved in the digestion and absorption of food. The zinc in red meat is much more easily absorbed than zinc from plants, grains and legumes. Beef contains 4.1 mg of zinc per 100 grams. Red meat is also rich in other important minerals like phosphorus, potassium, magnesium and selenium and the B vitamins, especially B12, B3 and B6 that help maintain nerve cells and normal blood formation.

Lean red meat helps reduce overall cholesterol in the blood in the same way as lean poultry and fish. Almost half of the fat in lean red meat is monounsaturated, the type of fat that helps lower blood cholesterol. Much of the saturated fat found in red meat is stearic acid, a form that doesn't raise blood cholesterol like other saturated fats do.

Red meat has been blamed for causing different types of cancer and clogging the arteries by raising cholesterol levels in the blood, but this is not true. The problem is that in the cultures where red meat is eaten as a component of high-carbohydrate diets, the above-mentioned diseases are common. In cultures where red meat is eaten mainly with vegetables and fruit, those diseases are not as common as they are in the modern westernized world. The most likely cause for these diseases is instead the high insulin level in the blood caused by overeating of carbohydrates, not red meat.

Myth number 11 - To stay in good health you have to drink 2 litres of water or more per day

In order to preserve health and proper functioning, the body should be hydrated at all times. Dehydration can cause many health problems, including a lack of minerals, cramps, kidney problems, loss of muscle tissue, blood pressure changes and more. The best way to keep the body hydrated during the day is to eat a balanced and healthy diet, rich in high water content foods like vegetables and fruit. High water content foods like vegetables and fruit also provide a lot of essential electrolytes that are necessary to keep water levels inside and outside of the cells in the proper balance.

The hype of drinking a lot of water during the day is an attempt to compensate for the lack of water in our modern diets, which are rich with processed foods that are dense in calories and low in water. Foods like breads, grains, pastas, cakes, sweets and others contain very little water and yet remain very dense in calories from carbohydrates. In most cases, the salt content is also very high in processed foods. Making these foods the bulk of our diet will cause dehydration, in addition to other unwanted health problems. Drinking a lot of tap water while on a diet made of concentrated foods can help a bit, but can also cause problems by forcing electrolytes out of the body. Mineral water may be a better choice, although it is devoid of fluorine (found in tap water). A combination of mineral and tap water can offer both benefits.

The amount of water that should be drunk daily for health benefits is very hard to estimate. People who rely on a healthy diet (rich in vegetables and fruit) will need less water on a daily basis, while people who rely on a diet rich in processed food will need to drink more water. People who are physically more active need more water than people who are not.

The best advice would be to eat a diet rich in high water content foods (vegetables and fruits) and drink water sensibly, whenever needed. Just guzzling litres of water because you have been advised that you need to drink "lots" of water can also be counterproductive. Eating unhealthily and trying to detoxify by drinking too many litres of water can still be damaging to your health. The powerful effects of an unhealthy diet cannot be eliminated simply by drinking extra water.

Myth number 12 - A low-calorie diet is the best way to lose weight

A low-calorie diet has been widely accepted as the best type of diet for weight loss. Although it is true that you will lose weight on a low-calorie diet, there are 2 major problems that make this type of diet only temporarily successful. First, not all of the weight lost on a low-calorie diet will come from fat — 50% of lost weight also comes from muscle tissue! Secondly, weight lost on a low-calorie diet is always regained within weeks and usually even more weight is gained after the low-calorie diet ends. Let's look at the reasons that create this problem with low-calorie diets.

On a low-calorie diet, although the body starts losing weight (50% of the loss from fat and 50% from muscle tissue), it also goes into starvation mode in order to preserve energy and continue functioning on the decreased intake of calories. In order to do that, the body has to slow down its own metabolism to lower the demand for calories. In order to slow down its metabolism, the body gets rid of its most metabolically active tissue: muscles. By getting rid of muscle tissue the body slows down its metabolism, thus requiring less overall energy for daily functioning. This is the reason why we lose 50% of muscle and 50% of fat on a low calorie diet. With the loss of muscle tissue and decreased metabolism, the body will significantly slow down its fat burning abilities. The longer we stay on a low-calorie diet, the less fat we will burn at the expense of muscle tissue.

Low-calorie diets also create cravings. The longer you stay on a low-calorie diet the stronger the cravings become. The day people give up the low-calorie diet they usually binge on enormous amounts of food which can continue for long periods. It may take days to satisfy and stop powerful cravings that may have developed over the period of weeks or months on a low-calorie diet. Once back on high-calorie binging, but with less muscle tissue then before starting the diet and now with a slower metabolism, the body will not be able to successfully process all these new calories and will immediately store most of them as fat. This is the reason why dieters, after giving up low-calorie diets, end up gaining more fat than they had before. Sound familiar?

Low-calorie diets are not the most effective way for losing extra body weight in the form of body fat. A balanced diet high in protein, vegetables and fruit in combination with weight training is the best way of permanently losing body fat while preserving efficient metabolism in the long run. Maintaining muscle mass through weight training will keep your metabolism high and burn mainly body fat whenever you try to lose weight.

The bottom line

- There are a lot of so called "myths" in nutrition that have done a lot of harm to people who have followed them.
- Some of the most popular myths are the ones that favour carbohydrates as the best food when it comes to fat loss.
- Another one that creates a lot of confusion is the myth about weight loss. Weight loss is totally irrelevant unless it only concerns the loss of fat. In the majority of cases where low-calorie,

high-carbohydrate diets are followed, weight loss is slightly attributable to fat loss, but primarily to the loss of muscle tissue.

- The protein scare is another myth that has devastated dieters by slowing down their metabolism through the loss of lean muscle tissue and the loss of muscle strength.
- Many other nutrition myths have been making life very hard for dieters. Unless the right information finds its way to the general public, nutrition myths will continue to do us harm.

The Ultimate Diet

Expectations are always extremely high when it comes to reliable advice about daily eating habits and the selection and amount of recommended foods that we should be eating. Everyone I have met throughout the decades of my involvement in sports and nutrition has expected a magic answer regarding the perfect diet, one that would help him or her to achieve a dream body and optimal health in record time. Consumer psychology is the same whether it comes to buying a mobile phone, car, sofa or nutritional advice. Once the price is paid for the service, regardless of the nature of the problem, expectations of perfect results are extremely high. The reality is that some products and services are instant and show their results immediately, whilst some advice and services simply require more time to deliver the expected results. One of these latter areas is definitely the world of nutrition. It usually takes months, and sometimes even years, to achieve results from nutritional programs and advice.

Nutritional changes are lifestyle changes and seldom get implemented right away. Very rarely have I had a client who has implemented all of my nutritional advice right away. Nutrition is a very delicate issue and the way an individual eats is influenced by many factors. We can argue about the importance of different factors, but there will always be influences like tradition, culture, religion, family, money, access to information, motivation, etc. I have to admit that when I come face to face with someone who has been eating certain types of food and following a certain diet for the last 40 years — while suffering badly from the same — my job to advise about the correct diet is far from easy. My advice is usually completely different from what may be expected and often disappointing for the client in terms of its implementation.

The ultimate diet is also not a seasonal experience; this is not a diet that will help you to get in shape for the summer holiday, or after a Christmas festive period. The ultimate diet is a part of your lifestyle and changes that are implemented in your way of eating should stay with you for the rest of your life. The ultimate diet should never be understood as a quick fix; it is rather a long-term commitment in implementing only natural foods in your daily diet and in your daily routine. Only as a part of a lifestyle change will the ultimate diet benefit you to its full potential.

Once you start on an ultimate diet, you will start benefiting from it instantly. Obvious changes that will show first include fat loss, energy increase, stronger immunity, quicker recovery, better ability to focus, higher motivation and improvement in overall well-being. The ultimate diet should also be followed by the ultimate weight training regime in order to optimise its potential. The ultimate diet, in cooperation with high intensity weight training, will help you to increase lean muscle mass, overall body strength and automatically lose fat.

The key answer to the ultimate solution, and hence the ultimate diet, is to understand our nature and identify the food that will help us to optimise our physical and intellectual human potential. Only foods that have been created by nature and have permitted us to have a life free from chronic diseases for most of our evolution can be the building blocks of the ultimate diet. We have, in previous chapters, identified what natural foods are, but the subject of this chapter will

be practical advice on implementing a daily diet that will successfully help the majority of the population. My own estimate is that no
more the 15% of the world population can respond positively to diets
rich in complex carbohydrates (grains). Giving a one-size-fits-all
solution that can satisfy every single person regarding healthy eating
is simply an impossible task. However, giving general guidance to
help everyone to identify their own individual characteristics, such
as metabolism, daily physical activity, glucose tolerance, insulin
sensitivity, daily caloric intake, etc., and create the best possible diet
and lifestyle practices is a much more realistic goal.

The ultimate diet is simply a way of communicating between the
individual and nature. Understanding that we are part of nature and
can only function properly while implementing the laws of nature
into our diet will help us to discover the simplest and most perfect
ways of eating. Our direct daily involvement in diets with the foods
that we are perfectly adapted to, and avoidance of the heavily processed edibles that have been and are still being invented daily by
man, not nature, is the cornerstone of what I have called the ultimate diet – the only right way of eating. The ultimate diet is not my
invention (it has been around for most of our evolution); it is simply
my understanding, recognition and reintroduction of the right diet
which will guarantee good health and freedom from chronic diseases.

The ultimate diet is also the only diet that will free energy trapped in
the heavy digestion of the wrong food, thereby strengthening immunity. People will also feel more physically energetic from following
the ultimate diet. Wrong diets, full of processed, denatured foods,
are simply a huge burden for the body; not only that the food has to
be digested, but also stored and eliminated. The harmful ingredients
of processed food are causing over-production of insulin, under-

production of glucagons, and they drain essential microelements from the body in order to be digested and absorbed. They increase cholesterol in the blood, cause build-up and calcification of cholesterol in the arteries, and at the same time slow down the transit time of the food through the digestive system, causing fermentation and putrefaction of macroelements and promotion of harmful bacteria. A huge amount of energy is used for the detoxification and unnecessary processing of useless ingredients introduced to the body by processed foods. That wasted energy manifests itself in a weakened immune system and less energy for other creative and productive life activities.

As we all know, there are essential elements (nutrients) which are only available from food and have to be ingested because we cannot produce (synthesise) them ourselves. As part of the focus of this chapter, we will concentrate on macronutrients and once again remind ourselves about the importance of essential amino acids and essential fatty acids. We have to obtain these essential components through our food since we cannot produce them ourselves, and remember, once again, there are no essential carbohydrates! Blood sugar (glucose), essential for all our activities and nourishment of the brain, can be produced from proteins, fats and ketones. In order to maintain a healthy blood sugar level, we actually don't have to eat any carbohydrates at all! They are simply not essential!

This basic fact of physiology has been heavily ignored and misinterpreted, allowing for the creation of unnatural diets that are high in carbohydrates. And although carbohydrates are present in almost all natural foods, they are present in the amounts that nature has perfectly measured for us. The amount of carbohydrates in fruit, vegetables, nuts and meats is far below the amount of carbohydrates in fake, commercially-made edibles. Not only the amount, but also the type of carbohydrates found in natural foods is such that it doesn't cause a high release of insulin and result in all the unhealthy side effects that this carries.

Natural foods, apart from containing essential amino and fatty acids, are also very high in water and fibre content, unlike the main staple foods of our modern era (starchy foods). The ultimate diet is the diet that offers high water content food, lots of necessary fibre and all the necessary essential amino and fatty acids.

The right proportion of proteins to carbohydrates to fat which has given me and most of my clients the best results in achieving impressive fat loss, whilst still retaining and even gaining new muscle tissue, has always been 40% - 40% - 20%. In cases of very slow metabolism and difficult fat loss, I have achieved great results with a proportion of 50% protein, 20% carbohydrates and 30% essential fats. The important fact to remember is that when carbohydrates are obtained from vegetables and fruit in order to achieve 20% or even 40% of daily caloric intake, a large amount of fibre and water is consumed at the same time. In combination with fibre and good fats as part of the ultimate diet, carbohydrates derived from vegetables and fruit are released slowly into the bloodstream, requiring less insulin production.

The ultimate diet is the only diet that also provides all necessary microelements like vitamins, minerals and trace elements. The proper balance of animal food (protein and fat) and plant food (fibres, carbohydrates, water, oils) provides a wide choice of natural sources of vitamins like B, A, C and others, and minerals like iron, magnesium, zinc, calcium and more. So far, there have been many other attempts to create a perfect diet. Unfortunately, in most other food strategies and recommended diets, the common scenario has been to underestimate or even exclude some of the major natural foods, denying access to essential micro and even macronutrients. I have had many clients who were completely disillusioned and demoralised, finding themselves in poor and unexpected physical shape after following many of the heavily promoted "popular" diets for a few months. Their defeat was always manifested in the following unwanted consequences: a loss of strength, loss of energy, lethargy, constant tiredness, loss of muscle mass and tone, a weak and unhealthy appearance, and sometimes a loss of weight but NOT FROM FAT. In almost all cases they regained all the lost weight and even gained more on top of that once the diet was over! Their look of desperation was always accompanied by the same response: "But I have done everything right, like it said in the book, and look at me now!"

All these undesired results that follow unnatural diets are always consequences of either overeating carbohydrates, overeating fat, under-eating protein (all coming from the wrong choice of food and wrong combination of food) or eating too little, as often advised by the "popular" nutrition books.

Sample menus

I will now provide a few different sample menus as part of the ultimate diet that should be considered as suggestions only. It's simply not possible to give a solution that will satisfy everyone, and individual variations will always have to be taken into consideration in order to establish the right amount of nutrients in every meal. It has always been expected of any nutrition book that it offer the right amount of food (nutrients) in every meal to satisfy every single individual. Every nutrition book that has tried to do that so far has got it wrong. It might seem like the perfect solution to recommend a nutrition strategy that would suit everyone perfectly, but when all the factors that determine the right diet for an individual are put together, we have a problem with one-size-fits-all scenarios. Factors such as gender, age, body weight, fitness level, metabolic efficiency, etc., all determine how much and what kind of food one should eat. Taking these into consideration, the only possible solution is to suggest guidelines that will help optimise the benefits of healthy eating for the general population.

For example, more physical activities on a daily basis (sports, heavy work, etc) demand more calories than an inactive lifestyle. A higher lean body weight requires more calories in order to keep all metabolic processes at their optimal levels. Younger people are metabolically more efficient and need more calories, and are capable of successfully managing more calories than older individuals whose metabolic processes are slower. Men need more calories (food) than women, simply because of their greater muscle mass and higher caloric expenditure. All these basic factors, as well as many others, shape every individual's diet regarding the amount of food and number of meals that should be eaten on a daily basis.

For a great majority of people, the choice and proportion of food that the ultimate diet provides will be the ideal solution. With the amount and proportion of macro and micronutrients, water content and high fibre presence, the food suggested in the ultimate diet will simply be the best possible choice.

There will always be people who require specific diets due to specific needs such as certain medical conditions, food intolerances or lowered digestive ability. Such individuals will have to follow diets prescribed to them by their medical professionals and they will have to consult their physicians before attempting any changes in the diets specifically created for them.

The number of meals in the ultimate diet varies from 3 to 6. Again, individuals with a higher caloric demand will need to eat more meals than individuals with lower caloric demand. I would not advise less than 3 meals per day to anyone, whilst 6 meals per day is the highest reasonable number of meals if a greater amount of food is required. Individuals with a slower metabolism process food more slowly and will require a lower number of meals, while individuals with higher metabolism who process food more quickly will need to eat a higher number of meals.

The size of the meals also depends on a few different factors and it should not be the same for everyone. Factors like gender, age, level of physical activity, intensity of weight training sessions, frequency of training, lean body size and metabolic speed will determine the size of the meals necessary for each individual. It would be totally wrong to advise eating the same size portions for everyone. The popular belief among fitness and nutrition professionals, that the body cannot absorb more than 30 grams of protein per single meal, is wrong and comes from having a limited understanding of human physiology and its metabolic processes. If this belief were true, we would all be more or less the same size and have the same level of strength, whilst there would be nobody like elite athletes, whose lean body weight often exceeds over 100 kilograms! They would probably starve eating only 30 grams of protein per meal. As yet more examples of how meal sizes vary, women usually eat less food per meal than men due to their lower body weight. Younger people tend to eat bigger meals than older people since they have a faster metabolism and more muscle mass. Inactive people eat less per single meal than people actively involved in sports due to their lower energy expenditures and slower metabolism. Individuals with higher lean body mass need more food per meal thanks to their higher need for proteins and other macro and micronutrients.

In some special instances, for example in the case of professional athletes, the number of meals can go even higher than 6. It's not unusual for top athletes to eat 8 or 9 meals per day. Heavyweight competitive bodybuilders, power-lifters, weight-lifters, swimmers, sprinters and other athletes involved in high-intensity sports are notorious for eating huge amounts of food and consuming high numbers of meals in order to maintain their muscle size while keeping body fat levels very low. More meals per day in combination with high-intensity training dramatically speeds up the metabolic processes in the body.

Sample menu 1

Meal 1: fruit and nuts
Meal 2: chicken and salad
Meal 3: fish and steamed vegetables
Meal 4: fruit and nuts
Meal 5: steak and salad

Sample menu 2

Meal 1: boiled eggs and cottage cheese
Meal 2: steak and steamed vegetables

Meal 3: fruit and nuts
Meal 4: fish and salad
Meal 5: mixed seafood salad
Meal 6: mixed salad and cold turkey cuts

Sample menu 3

Meal 1: liver and boiled eggs
Meal 2: fish, salad and nuts
Meal 3: fruit
Meal 4: meat and steamed vegetables

Things to remember:

1. Eat raw (fresh) fruit and vegetables.
2. If you steam your vegetables, keep them crunchy and don't over-cook them.
3. Eat nuts raw, not roasted or salted.
4. Use olive or flax seed oil in your salads.
5. Never cook in oils or expose oils to high temperature.
6. Don't overcook your meat and fish.
7. Eat low-fat dairy products like yoghurt and cottage cheese only if you have no lactose intolerance.
8. Avoid milk.
9. Never overeat; leave the table once you have satisfied your hunger, not when you reach the feeling of fullness.
10. Wait until you are a bit hungry before you have a meal, don't let time be your guide as when to eat, and let your instincts and slight hunger decide when the right time is for the next meal.

11. Take your supplements daily, especially if exercising regularly.
12. Three crucial supplements that should not be missed are fish oil, vitamin C and vitamin E.

The bottom line:

- Like all other species, humans should eat food that has been designed for them by nature.
- We all have built-in instincts that signal us when it's time to eat and which food is the best choice. Once these instincts are awakened again, with the help of the ultimate diet, it will be easy to continue to eat healthily.
- The ultimate diet is the diet that suggests natural food in the right amount and right proportion.
- Processed foods have no place in the ultimate diet.
- The ultimate diet offers the perfect amount and combination of all essential macro and micronutrients.
- The ultimate diet will help eliminate the bad consequences caused by eating the wrong food while preserving good health and strong immunity.
- In order to benefit from the ultimate diet, every individual will have to assess their own daily energy expenditure and energy needs and then follow the suggestions from the ultimate diet in order to establish the right amount and proportion of food for them, as well as the right number of meals per day.

Exercise

Physical exercise deserves coverage in every book about nutrition. Although I devote much more attention to this subject in my exercise books, we still have to be reminded about the importance of exercise in connection to healthy eating and living. The body needs quality nutrients in the right balance on a consistent daily basis in order to function properly. It also needs daily exercise that has to be intense enough and last long enough to promote its optimal functioning.

Our bodily systems are all inter-related and work in synergy. The health and strength of all bodily systems can be directly influenced through our muscular system, which is the only system that can be controlled voluntarily. By engaging our muscular system in different physical activities, like exercise, we indirectly engage our respiratory, vascular, lymphatic, cardiac, skeletal, endocrine and digestive systems. With regular engagement in intense exercise, apart from strengthening skeletal muscle tissue, we also strengthen our lungs, heart, bones, and arteries, improve digestion and elimination and balance our hormones. Engaging our bodily systems through exercise results in more efficient metabolic processes which are directly linked to the food that we eat.

The phrase that we have all heard many times, "you are what you eat", is only partially true. The reality is actually "you are what you absorb". You can have two people eating the same food and one of them can end up being in good health and shape, while the other one can end up being out of shape and in bad health. The same food eaten by different people will not guarantee the same outcome. The final outcomes of good health and physical shape are not only influenced by eating properly, but also by many other different factors. Eating is one thing while absorbing the same food is something very different.

The rate of absorption and amount of nutrients that get absorbed by the body also depend greatly on the physical activity of an individual. The threshold of absorption of macro and micronutrients changes with the metabolic demands initiated by intense physical engagement (sports). People who are actively involved in sports need higher amounts of protein, fat, carbohydrates (from fruit and vegetables), vitamins and minerals than inactive people. Therefore they will also absorb more nutrients thanks to the increased demand for them.

A typical example of increased absorption due to a higher demand can be demonstrated with the mineral calcium. As long as an individual is physically active (in sports), the amount of lean muscle mass will be relatively high. Bigger and stronger muscles will force the body to create and maintain strong and healthy bones by absorbing more calcium and storing it in the bones. All the calcium in the world would not improve deteriorating bones and their calcium loss unless the demand for stronger bones was created through intense exercise. This is one of many examples that show how physical exercise influences the destiny of healthy food in the body and how it complements nutrition.

Another example regarding the same issue is the protein demand in physically active vs. inactive people. For years, nutritionists who advocated high-carbohydrate diets tried to convince the world that athletes (and others involved in regular sports activities) needed the same amount of protein as physically inactive people. They tried to justify this theory by pointing to the protein absorption threshold. Their view was that nobody could absorb more than 30 grams of protein in a single meal! I have never come across any scientific proof for this nonsense. But what I have come across time and time again during my 30 years of active involvement in sports and nutrition is that athletes do eat much more than 30 grams of protein per meal! An average meal eaten by an athlete contains no less than 50 grams of protein and up to a staggering 100 grams! I have never seen an athlete eating a meal and restricting himself to a ridiculous amount of only 30 grams of protein! In the real world, people do eat more protein than has been suggested by the "experts".

The reason for this "adequate" amount of protein (more than 30 grams) in physically active people is simply the higher need for muscle and tissue repair created by the intensity of exercise, and amino acids (protein components) are the most important ingredients needed for the repair of muscle tissue. Although inactive people don't need as much protein as athletes, in my experience I still don't feel that they eat enough quality protein. Skin problems, bad nails and hair, weakness in the muscles and constant tiredness are only some of the very heavy consequences of high quality protein deficiency.

Regular exercise also creates a healthy hunger, a hunger for essential nutrients, not just for the calories (carbohydrates and saturated fats). Everyone actively involved in intense sports would agree that nothing is more satisfying than a steak or chicken meal after an intense training session. Physical engagement demands adequate food in order to rebuild and replenish emptied stores and burned tissue. Healthy hunger, as I like to call it, can only be induced by proper exercise. If I could wrap it all up in a single sentence, regular exercise will help you to instinctively seek the right nutritious food, to better digest your healthy food and most importantly, to help you absorb the essential nutrients in an amount and rate that would not be possible without regular exercise.

Things to remember:

1. Exercise regularly 4 - 6 times per week.
2. Concentrate on high intensity exercises like weight lifting, sprinting, swimming, etc.
3. If you want to do lower intensity exercises like power walking, cycling, running, etc., do them as interval training, changing intensity during their performance.
4. Incorporate regular exercise as a part of your lifestyle.

The bottom line

- Physical exercise complements healthy eating; good health and fat loss are much more easily achieved when exercise and healthy eating are implemented together.
- Physical exercise creates a higher demand for nutrients and therefore results in their better absorption.

Your Shopping Basket

One of the very common questions that I get asked almost daily from people interested in healthy living is: "Ok, now that I know what is good and what is bad for me, what should be on my shopping list?"

Everybody would agree that entering the supermarket or farmers' market is the true nutrition reality test where correct choices need to be made. We can leave the market with a basket full of goodness or a basket full of junk. Buying the right food is very important since the presence of the wrong food in our homes easily triggers temptations to eat them. We all know what happens with the box of chocolates that someone kindly brought us as a present, or with a big tub of ice cream that our guests bought for us...

On the next few pages, I provide a list of suggested food items that you should find room for in your shopping basket and a list of food items that you should stay away from.

Foods to eat - protein and fat sources

Fish	**Poultry**	**Fermented low-fat dairy products**
Salmon	Chicken	
Tuna	Turkey	Yoghurt
Mackerel	Ostrich, etc	Cottage cheese
Haddock		Low-fat cheese, etc.
Sardines	**Meat (lean cuts)**	
Herring	Beef	
Cod	Pork	
Sea Bass	Lamb	
Monkfish	Venison	
Swordfish, etc.	Bison, etc.	
Seafood	**Eggs**	
Scallops		
Squid	**Internal Organs**	
Octopus	Liver	
Crab	Heart	
Prawns	Kidneys	
Oysters		
Mussels, etc.		

Foods to eat - carbohydrate and fibre sources

Fruits	Vegetables	Oils and Fibre (Nuts)
Apples	Lettuce	Almonds
Pears	Cabbage	Hazelnuts
Figs	Mushrooms	Walnuts
Plums	Green leaves	Brazil nuts
Apricots	Carrots	Cashew nuts
Peaches	Spinach	Pecan nuts
Grapes	Onions	Pistachios
Pineapple	Garlic	Macadamia nuts, etc.
Oranges	Leeks	
Grapefruits	Parsnips	**Oils**
Cherries	Celery	Olive oil
Strawberries	Broccoli	Flax seed oil
Raspberries	Cauliflower	Sunflower oil
Blueberries	Brussels sprouts	Almond oil
Blackberries	Artichokes	Avocado oil
Bananas	Asparagus	Safflower oil
Mangoes	Aubergines	Fish oil, etc.
Papaya	Courgettes, etc.	
Melon		
Watermelon	**Vegetable fruits**	
Kiwi, etc.	Tomatoes	
	Peppers	
	Cucumber	
	Avocado	

Food to avoid - protein and fat sources

Fatty meats

Fatty pork cuts

Fatty lamb cuts

Fatty beef cuts

Others

Tinned meats

Tinned fish

Dried or salted meat

Dried or salted fish

All processed meats and
meat products

All processed fish and
fish products

Milk

Food to avoid - carbohydrate sources

Starchy foods

Potatoes

Sweet potatoes

Oats, rice, etc.

All starchy food

Processed foods

Bread

Pasta

Pastries

Pizza and others

All processed foods
made of flours

All processed meats and
meat products

Processed foods

All processed fish and
fish products

All dried fruits

Raisins

Dried apricots

Dried figs, etc.

Fat and oil sources

Animal fat

Saturated processed oils

Hydrogenated fats

Sugars

White sugar

Brown sugar

Fructose

Corn syrup

Maple syrup

Honey and others

**All foods and drinks
made of sugars**

Cakes

Sweets

Ice Cream

Chocolate

Biscuits

Sugared juices

Sugared fizzy drinks

It is obvious that the healthiest option is to eat food in its natural, wholesome, fresh state. Everything that nature created for human consumption in its raw, natural shape is a perfect food. Fruits, vegetables, nuts and seeds should always be eaten raw, without cooking, freezing or drying them. By cooking fruits and vegetables, their alkalinity changes and they become acidic, delivering a completely opposite effect on human health.

Although fish and meat can also be eaten raw (steak tartar, sushi, etc.) today's modern farming with its necessary food production technology can hardly guarantee the safety of raw meat and fish for consumption. However, meat and fish should not be overcooked, in order to preserve their nutrients at the highest levels possible.

Everything that cannot be eaten in its natural state (like grains, pulses and legumes) and that has to be heavily processed in order to be sold commercially, has inflicted the health miseries that we know today. For example, all the products made from flour, such as bread, pasta, cereals, cakes, pastries and others, are the major cause of all chronic diseases due to their processed nature and unique ability to greatly increase blood sugar levels and trigger a high release of insulin into the bloodstream.

The bottom line

- Fresh food (vegetables, fruits, meat, fish, etc.) is the only food that should end up in your shopping basket.
- Do not buy processed food or food that has a long shelf life (pasta, rice, frozen food, sweets, tinned food, etc.). Natural foods have a very short shelf life.

15 Tips for Effective Fat Loss

These fundamental tips that I will now offer you are not based only on theories. They have been personally learned by me, first hand, during my own long experience with fat loss. Besides the fact that I had to reduce my own body fat levels down to some 5 - 6% for competitive reasons (something I have had to repeat 46 times for 46 bodybuilding competitions), I have also had to use the same principles for thousands of my clients with amazing results in fat loss over a period of more than two decades.

As you should have now realised, I don't talk about weight loss in my books and articles, I always talk about fat loss! Weight loss is relatively easy to achieve. All you need to do is to go on low-calorie diet (which I like to call a starvation diet) and fight your way through. Some people will lose more weight and some people will lose less weight over periods of 6 - 10 weeks or more. The one thing that they will all have in common though is the constant struggle to stay on the low-calorie diet and fight all kinds of food cravings.

This constant battle against starvation will always end up with the same result. Once enough weight has been lost and the target weight has been achieved, the pleasure of stopping the low-calorie diet will culminate in repeated binging that will last as long as it is necessary for the body to regain the weight that was lost — and even add extra new weight! A battle fought using low calorie-diets aimed at WEIGHT LOSS is a battle that you will always lose in the long run!

Why does this happen? Why is it that weight lost on a low-calorie diet always has to come back and extra weight always piles on? The answer to this is very simple and lies in our physiology. The body is more than happy to lose extra body fat. Any other weight loss, mainly from muscle tissue, is the last thing that our body likes. Muscle tissue is the tissue that is responsible for movement, mobility, bone density, healthy functioning of the cardiac, vascular, respiratory, digestive and other systems in the body. Therefore, muscle tissue is much more important to our overall health and well-being than is commonly believed. At the same time, since muscle tissue has a prolific blood supply, its metabolic rate is much higher in absolute terms than the metabolic rate of fat tissue. During periods of low-calorie dieting, weight loss accounts for an average loss of 50% body fat and 50% muscle tissue. This is the problem that advocates of low-calorie diets and people who only talk about WEIGHT LOSS don't understand and therefore cannot solve.

To make matters even worse, loss of muscle tissue induced by a period of starvation (low-calorie dieting) causes the overall metabolism to slow down. When the dieter reaches their targeted weight, although having lost body weight, they will also have slowed down their metabolism dramatically and all new weight gain (which will ultimately occur) will be composed of 100 % body fat! What actually happens in most of the cases of low-calorie diets is that you can expect to end up fatter than you were before you started dieting!

Once again, it is fat loss that matters, not weight loss. Losing only body fat is not an easy process. It requires at least a basic understanding of physiology, the metabolic processes, nutrition, exercise and requires enough motivation to implement all of the necessary changes into your lifestyle.

It is very interesting that "experts" who advise people on low-calorie diets also tend not to talk much about the importance of exercise in fat loss, or at best only advise a moderate amount of low-intensity exercise (known incorrectly as aerobic or cardiovascular exercise) a few times per week. The absence of exercise or the practice of low-intensity exercise only is totally counterproductive for the purpose of fat loss! Exercise benefits fat loss only when it is directly related to maintaining or building new muscle mass. Muscles, being the most metabolically demanding tissues, consume more fuel (energy) and are directly responsible for fat loss. Less muscle mass means less fat loss, more muscle mass means more fat loss. Inactivity or engaging in low-intensity, long duration exercises only is the best way to lose muscle mass while dieting and slowing down our overall metabolic efficiency! The only way to preserve muscle tissue while trying to lose body fat is to implement high-intensity weight training 4 - 6 times per week! Any other type of exercise apart from high-intensity weight training will not only be useless, but also counter-productive.

15 Tips

Tip 1: Mathematical calorie counting and calorie reduction are not the only things that matter. Let proper food selection take care of the right amount of calories that you consume and this will help you lose fat.

Tip 2: Choose only natural foods like fruits and vegetables and eat them fresh and raw. Fish and meat should not be overcooked. Natural foods are very low in calories so don't bother counting them.

Tip 3: Eat only when you are hungry. By eating fresh natural food you will end up eating only a few times per day, each time triggered by the sensation of slight hunger rather than a preconceived time-table. There is no rule that determines how long you have to wait between meals. Different lifestyles, activity levels and metabolic rates will create different durations needed to digest food in the first stage and get the body ready for the next meal.

Tip 4: Don't snack between meals. Proper meals need time to be digested and every snack added between meals while digestion is still taking place will disrupt and slow down digestion.

Tip 5: Try to eat the same size meals throughout the day. Eating bigger and then smaller meals is not the best way to optimally digest and absorb food.

Tip 6: Avoid eating late at night. During sleep your digestion and metabolism slow down and most of the energy from food gets stored as fat, whilst the body also doesn't burn much energy.

Tip 7: Make sure that most of your meals are made of protein and vegetables. Eat fruit on its own some 30 minutes before meals.

Tip 8: Never attempt diets that are very low in fat or fat-free. Use natural cold-pressed oils in your salads and supplement your diet with fish oil. Eating essential fats will actually help you to burn more unwanted body fat.

Tip 9: Eat sensibly. Once your hunger is gone and you feel satisfied, you should stop eating. Do not continue eating until you get full. The difference between being satisfied and being full can be up to 1 500 calories in one meal!

Tip 10: Supplement your diet with all essential minerals, vitamins and microelements. Always take your supplements after meals.

Tip 11: Never eat empty calories found in processed foods like sweets, cakes, biscuits, chocolates, bread, pasta, etc. Foods made of sugar, flour and saturated fats are the ones that most contribute to making you fat.

Tip 12: Be active. Use the stairs instead of the lift. Walk whenever possible, rather than drive. Don't avoid housework and gardening. Being more active in general will help you lose fat and stay lean.

Tip 13: Make resistance (weight) training your number one priority. Train with weights 4 - 5 times per week. High-intensity weight training is the only type of training that will stimulate fat loss, not just weight loss, up to 24 hours after your session! The increased metabolic activity that results after weight training will burn your body fat even during resting hours. By adding extra pounds of lean muscle you will burn even more calories each day from body fat.

Tip 14: If you still want to perform low-intensity, long-duration activities (that are not very efficient in burning body fat), choose the safest ones like swimming and fast walking. Even with these types of exercises, your best bet again is to increase the intensity of the exercise through fast swimming or uphill walking.

Tip 15: Incorporate exercise into your lifestyle and do it on a regular basis. Getting in shape should not just be a seasonal goal (like prior to a holiday or after Christmas). Once you get in shape, you should stay in shape for good. This is only possible if exercise becomes a part of your daily routine and an integral part of your new lifestyle.

Sports Nutrition

Sports nutrition is a very delicate science. Athletes and highly active individuals comprise a sector of the population that deserves special attention when it comes to proper nutrition. Physically active people burn more calories, and people involved in serious sports activities also burn more muscle tissue during training sessions and sports events than the rest of the population. Stressed muscle tissue needs to recover adequately and be ready for new training sessions and new activities. Unless recovery and rebuilding of the involved muscles and connective tissues occurs, every future effort will be compromised and the risk of injuries will increase. It is not only athletes in high-intensity sports such as bodybuilding, weight lifting, sprinting, swimming, gymnastics or wrestling that need a specific nutrition regime, but also endurance athletes like long-distance runners, cyclists, long-distance swimmers and others.

Higher levels of muscle damage result from partaking in higher intensity sports and this leads to a need for more high quality protein to rebuild the muscle tissues. Long-duration sports activities expend more energy that needs to be replaced, so more high quality energy foods are then needed (fats and carbohydrates). In both types of sports, essential minerals and vitamins are a must and have to be supplemented accordingly.

Throughout my many years of involvement in competitive sports, I have met many athletes from different sports disciplines. What I have learned from my own experience and that of others is that athletes are very much involved in nutrition and would try anything in order to give their bodies the best possible combination of macro and micronutrients. In this constant striving for perfect nutrition, too many of them, unfortunately, make mistakes favouring some macro-nutrients or micronutrients at the expense of others. The favourite macronutrients are always protein and carbohydrates, and many athletes simply focus on them too much in their daily diets. It is common that some of them, especially athletes that are interested in muscle growth, eat the same high protein food day after day, while completely ignoring fats and carbohydrates. There are also others who constantly eat high-carbohydrate meals day after day instead, neglecting protein and fats.

I have met very few people who have understood the importance of proper food combination and balanced supplementation. It is almost a rule that essential fats never find their place even in the diets of elite athletes! Essential fats are a nonexistent term in the vocabulary of most people seriously involved in sports.

Minerals and vitamins are also unfamiliar territory for many athletes. Most of the athletes I have met are usually heavily focused on vita-mins C and E, while neglecting the importance of vitamins like D and B12, for example. Calcium is the most popular mineral amongst ath-letes, while magnesium and zinc for example rarely get consideration.

On the next few pages, I identify a few critical problem areas that are common in athlete nutrition and have caused a lot of problems in their careers resulting in injuries, common infections, loss of strength or endurance before and during events, slowed progress, weight problems and lack of confidence.

Problem areas for athletes:

1. Lack of the essential fats in the diet.
2. Over-consumption of carbohydrates at the expense of protein and essential fats.
3. Over-consumption of protein at the expense of fats and carbohydrates.
4. Low and/or unbalanced intake of minerals and vitamins.
5. Lack of fibre.
6. Over-reliance on protein supplements at the expense of natural protein sources.
7. Obsession with energy drinks.
8. Crash diets in order to achieve a target weight.

1. Lack of essential fats in the diet

Whilst most of the attention goes towards carbohydrates and protein in athletes' diets, essential fats have been heavily neglected. The essential fatty acids found in fish oil and flax seed oil, for example, are essential for optimal health, muscle and organ tissue function, and higher energy levels. They improve the absorption of other nutrients relevant to muscle strength and growth as well as for energy production. In order to obtain enough "good" fats, athletes should eat more fish containing omega-3 fatty acids (salmon, tuna, mackerel and others), more grass-fed beef, and should use more fish oil, flax seed oil, and olive oil. In controlled amounts, the natural unrefined animal fats found in eggs, lean cuts of pork, beef and lamb are also good sources of essential fatty acids.

2. Over-consumption of carbohydrates at the expense of protein and essential fats

It is not uncommon that athletes often neglect protein and fat intake while over-consuming carbohydrates, in the belief that carbohydrates will give them more energy necessary for athletic performance. There is a common belief that complex carbohydrates are good for you. Apart from the manufacturers of grain products, there is no one else who will benefit from this misinformation. Carbohydrates, simple or complex, all turn into glucose, triggering high amounts of insulin to be produced in order to be delivered to the muscle and fat cells. The high production of insulin will cause a blood sugar roller coaster causing a string of health problems, and more importantly for athletes, a drop in energy. Yes, more carbohydrates in your diet will actually make you less energetic! Due to insulin, the energy gained from high-carbohydrate foods will be lowered below normal levels within a very short time. Balanced diets with controlled and selected amounts of carbohydrates are the best way to keep athletes in top shape and with constantly available energy for athletic performance.

3. Over-consumption of carbohydrates at the expense of protein and essential fats

Over-consumption of protein is very common among strength athletes and bodybuilders. In a constant struggle to get stronger and bigger, these athletes are known to overeat protein whether in food or in the form of protein supplements. In reality, it is very difficult to over-eat protein from animal sources such as beef, chicken, pork or fish. The human body has its own mechanisms to stop us eating protein-rich food once we reach the optimum amount of protein that can be successfully digested and absorbed. It is only possible to digest and absorb extra amounts of protein through protein drinks on top of high amounts of food-based protein. Although by utilising this approach athletes may ensure that they are not going to miss out on the necessary protein needed to grow new muscle tissue, there will be other important nutrients missed. Inadequate intake of fats and carbohydrates will slow down progress and cause unwanted health consequences. A properly balanced diet in which every macronutrient has its place is essential for long-term success and good health.

4. Low and/or unbalanced intake of minerals and vitamins

I was very surprised to find that lots of athletes are simply not eating enough fresh vegetables and fruits, while some of them are not eating them at all! This crucial mistake is unfortunately denying them access to essential minerals and vitamins in combination with necessary enzymes that are found only in fresh, uncooked and unprocessed plant foods.

Regarding vitamin and mineral supplements, unbalanced intake is still common among many athletes; simply taking one or two multi-vitamin and mineral tablets a day is not enough. Apart from this, there are also very important extra vitamins C (up to 3 - 4 grams), E (up to 800 IU), calcium, chromium, magnesium, zinc and others that will never be possible to squeeze into a single tablet or two simply because of the sheer quantity needed. The correct amount of all the micronutrients are outlined in the previous chapters.

Vitamins and minerals are crucial for so many of the biochemical processes in the body. For athletes' best interest in preventing injuries, protecting them from poor digestion and nutrient assimilation, and gaining maximum amounts of strength, speed and stamina, micronutrients from food and selected supplements have to be available in their correct amount and proper balance.

5. Lack of fibre

A lack of vegetables, fruits and nuts in a daily diet usually results in a lack of fibre. A lack of fibre can cause constipation and also deposition of different substances in the linings of the stomach and small and large intestines, therefore decreasing the absorption of nutrients. Having enough fibre in athletes' diets is another reason why adequate amounts of fresh fruits and vegetables have to be incorporated on a regular basis. Raw nuts are also a great source of fibre and they should be eaten on a daily basis.

6. Over-reliance on protein supplements at the expense of natural protein sources

The common euphoria about the importance of drinking protein shakes has taken over every single gym around the globe. More and more people are convinced that if you really want to get in shape and gain some muscles while losing body fat, the best and only way to do it is to drink 2, 3 or more protein shakes every day! I was also one of the followers of this "great" idea and in my early days of weight training, I also believed that at least 3 protein shakes needed to be taken daily in order to make a serious change. This of course affected the number of meals I ate, which had to adjust around the "essential" protein shakes. Nowadays protein shakes are much better tasting and are made from much better ingredients than some 25 years ago. But although the quality is much better than before, protein shakes should only remain supplements in athletes' diets and never be substituted for meals made from real natural food. It is wrong to believe that extra strength, speed and muscle size can only be achieved with the help of protein shakes. Top achievements in all sports are possible with natural food only and without a single drop of a protein shake! Use them sparingly and only when there is no time to eat the real stuff. Convenience is the best thing that protein shakes can provide you.

7. Obsession with energy drinks

Energy drinks are yet another type of product that have found a place in the everyday lives of many athletes. It is a common belief that energy drinks will help all athletes during their training sessions or competitions. The truth is that the energy you use during physical training sessions mainly comes from the glycogen (stored carbohydrates) in your muscles and liver and, in the long run, from body fat. Glycogen used in sports activities is stored the day before your training session and it is important to regularly eat properly in order to keep your glycogen stores full at all times. Sugary drinks full of different acids (phosphoric acid, citric acid, and others), artificial flavouring, sweeteners and artificial colouring are no match for natural food when it comes to energy replacement. If you drink common energy drinks you should be aware that your body needs to work harder in order to manage and eliminate all of these artificial substances, wasting a lot of energy in the process that can instead be used for sports activities.

8. Crash diets in order to achieve a target weight

Crash diets are not only popular among the general population but also among athletes. In order to lose substantial amounts of weight in a short period of time (a week or two), people put themselves on crash diets. Because of the very small amount of food (calories) eaten on these types of diets, body weight drops dramatically in a relatively short time. Unfortunately, most of the weight lost that way comes from water loss. Muscles, being composed of 70% water, are the first tissues to suffer from this heavy loss. Body fat is the second source of lost weight and it is estimated that 60% or more of the weight lost during crash diets comes from the muscles! Muscle tissue should be the last tissue lost during any type of diet, so going on a crash diet should never be an option for you.

Once significant amounts of muscle tissue are lost due to a crash diet, strength levels drop immediately, as do speed, endurance and a winning attitude. Being the most metabolically active tissue, loss of muscle also leads ultimately to a slowdown in overall metabolism, which in turn leads to faster fat accumulation and the weight that always returns after crash diets are finished is usually weight gained from new fat! Plan your competitions a few months in advance and if you need to lose some body weight due to a target class weight, adjust your diet accordingly using my advice about healthy eating from previous chapters.

The bottom line:

- Athletes have different nutritional requirements than inactive people. The higher the intensity of a particular sport, the more protein is required.
- Although athletes generally pay a lot of attention to nutrition, they still make a lot of mistakes by over-eating particular macro-nutrients or under-eating others.

- The right balance of essential macronutrients in the diet is more important than the amount of a particular macronutrient.
- The most over-eaten macronutrients among athletes are carbohydrates and protein.
- Supplements are often over-relied upon in sports nutrition and often used to replace real, fresh food. This is a big mistake since protein powders and other ergogenic aids cannot replace the importance and power of natural food.

What Does the Future Hold?

Eating regularly and in enough quantity is a major concern of all living species on our planet. Our fellow mammals spend all their lives in constant search for food, and when they fail to find it they simply vanish. Food has never been guaranteed and the lives of all living organisms have evolved around a daily struggle to find proper and sufficient food. In order to survive, every species has had to change their anatomy and physiology; they have had to adapt. In some cases animals' necks have become longer, or the overall body size has changed, while some have changed their skin colour, or become shorter or taller. In our case, humans have introduced tools, discovered agriculture, improved technology and managed to produce enough food to feed ourselves in a way that we have never done before. More available food has enabled the development of larger and more abundant human societies. Life conditions have become much better and the world population has skyrocketed to an amazing 6 billion. The continuous and increased production of food around the world is the key factor in helping the development of civilisation at an unprecedented pace. Human civilisation has moved forward much faster in the last 10 000 years than it has done in the millions of years before then.

The critical stage in our evolution was reached with the discovery of agriculture. With the introduction of grains into our diet, we became able for the first time in our history to preserve and store food (grains) for longer periods and eat it whenever it was needed. Our feeding experience until then was very different — food had to be eaten right away after killing or picking, since hunters and gatherers could not preserve their food for as long as agricultural communities could. With more certainty about nutrition and life security, societies also had more time to devote to developing new technology and building more sustainable houses, bridges, roads, aqueducts, reservoirs, etc., and civilisation started taking off. Improved life conditions thanks to agriculture allowed humans to multiply in the billions. However, even though the human race dramatically improved in terms of numbers, the quality of life didn't necessarily follow at the same pace. Although everything looked great thanks to the development of agriculture, grains were not as innocent as a lot of us would have liked to believe.

The introduction of grains into our diet has simply changed the human menu for good. Grains were not just added to a diet that until then only knew meat, vegetables and fruits, but they have quickly TAKEN OVER our diet. Being much cheaper to produce and to buy, grains simply pushed meat, vegetables and fruit out of the top positions in our everyday diets. This legacy of grains has continued until today. Foods that had once been staple items became the least eaten foods in western societies (and other societies as well). The old, traditional foods of hunters and gathers, like vegetables, and then fruit, followed by fish and meat have lost the game against grain-derived foods.

Refined grains have brought a lot of calories with them, but these calories are mainly empty ones, without quality protein, or essential minerals and vitamins. They have also caused widespread malnutrition of essential food elements like amino acids, vitamins, minerals, trace elements, essential fatty acids and enzymes. And although people have become heavier, bigger and fatter, they have also started suffering from essential food component deficiency.

Carrying a lot of easily digestible calories found in all kinds of flour, sugars and alcohol, grains have caused something completely new for humans throughout evolution: chronic disease. Although armed with an extremely capable but also heavily overworked organ — the pancreas — humans are still losing the battle against diseases triggered by hyperproduction of insulin. The hormone directly linked with most chronic diseases and indirectly with all of them, insulin has been forced in huge amounts into most of our bloodstreams. Thanks to grains, we have developed the x syndrome that is now the officially recognised name for all chronic diseases caused by hyperproduction of insulin.

While the scientific world and pharmaceutical industry pretend to be the saviours of the human race (they are pushing hard to develop the new miracle medications that will eliminate the consequences of over-eating of grains and grain-made products), it seems that there is still no effort from the governments to limit the consumption of grains and try to bring people closer to the foods that nature has created for humans. This kind of effort would cost much less and would definitely help people live healthier lives.

So, the question that we as a human race are facing nowadays is: what awaits us in the future? Is it going to be a future where we will enjoy freedom from chronic diseases, or a time when we will master the science of replacing organs and easily eliminating the consequences of diseases which will be considered more or less normal?

If we look at eating patterns over the last century, the one thing that many cultures around the world have in common is overeating. In the case of the western world, the amount of food that people have eaten has steadily increased from one decade to another. The increase in food consumption perfectly correlates with technological progress in food production. Crops are produced more quickly, more cheaply and are now available to anyone, anywhere and at very low cost. People are eating more sugars and grain products than ever before. Processed grains and sugars, and the products made from them, have enabled people to consume huge amounts of calories, many times more than those eaten in the past.

Comparing the amount of calories in processed food to the amount in natural foods clearly demonstrates the fundamental difference, which is the major cause of chronic diseases. The calories found in two slices of toast equal the amount of calories found in one kilogram of broccoli! An average portion of pasta contains the same amount of calories as three kilograms of tomatoes! I hope that by now it's clear to everyone that it is impossible to overeat natural food and the calories found within. Overeating is always related to denatured processed foods and malnutrition of essential macro and micronutrients. Natural food is full of essential micro and macronutrients and never associated with malnutrition and overeating. Natural foods contain macronutrients in the amounts and types that do not cause hyperproduction of insulin like processed foods do.

Well, one might ask, what then stands between existing eating habits, which are causing so much health misery, and the healthy food choices that could completely reverse the health situation in the developed world, i.e. eliminate self-inflicted chronic diseases?

For a reasonable person the answer should be straightforward: the problem, once identified, should then be eliminated and replaced with a different and well thought-out approach. Once the problem has been identified and the answer has been offered, the remaining question is: do we have results? Are we improving the health situation which is directly related to the food we eat?

As usually happens, it takes time to change habits imposed by tradition, religion, ignorance and lack of knowledge. But things can be improved and we can take control of chronic diseases. Once we understand the causes of chronic diseases, it is much easier to start implementing changes.

The changes needed to improve the current health situation have to be implemented from the very beginning of a child's upbringing and in the first stages of education. Children have to be taught what natural food is, what the benefits of eating fresh, raw fruit and vegetables, meat and fish are and what the risks of eating processed foods full of sugars and carbohydrates, salt, additives and artificial colouring and flavourings are. Education is the first step and also the first stage of productive change that will help us improve our health situation. Without education from a very early stage it is simply impossible to achieve any long-term positive changes. Once healthy eating habits have been built, they have to continue as part of a healthy lifestyle to maintain the expected results. Unless a new nutritional approach is fully incorporated into one's lifestyle, it will never generate enough power and consistency over the long term.

There are also other factors that can support and help a new nutritional approach stay on course as a part of a new lifestyle. Factors such as regular exercise, a positive mental attitude and a balanced everyday lifestyle (business, social and private life) go hand in hand with healthy eating. Unless all these factors are incorporated into a new lifestyle, any change adopted by the majority of the western population will not result in a significant change in the current health situation. Insulin resistance will continue to dominate as the cause of deadly chronic diseases.

So, for everyone who is interested in a good quality of life, healthy eating, regular exercise, a positive attitude, balanced life and the challenges of love and friendship are the things that have to be made a priority and implemented.

The future of the species depends on the engagement of its own individuals. Unless the majority of individuals take it upon themselves to change, the species as a whole will not change or benefit from a new approach. In a way, our own individual destiny is not only ours, but also belongs to the collective self, to the human species itself. And as long as we understand ourselves as a part of this species, our individual efforts to implement positive changes will contribute both to the improvement of the species and the individual.

The bottom line

- Since grains have pushed natural food out of people's everyday diet, chronic diseases have skyrocketed.
- Fresh natural food like vegetables, fruit, meat and fish can offer a way out of the modern health crisis.
- Healthy eating should be part of lifestyle change that will guarantee long-term good quality of life.

Also from Nash Jocic:

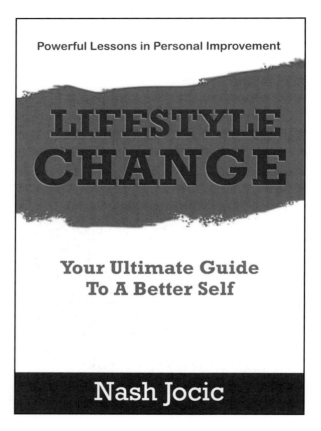

More Books:

"Weight Training for Men"

"Fat Loss"

For more info see: www.ultimateshape.com

DVDs:

7 Training DVDs for Men

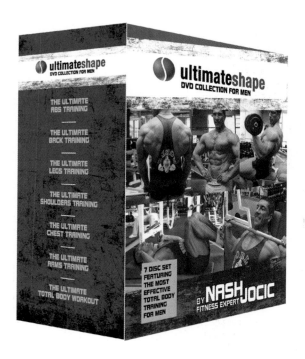

For more info see: www.ultimateshape.com

DVDs:

4 Training DVDs for Women

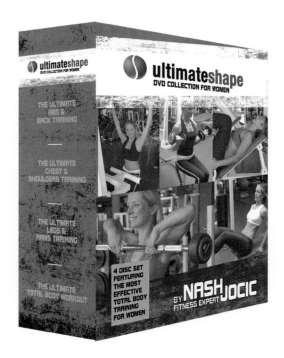

For more info see: www.ultimateshape.com

Notes:

Notes:

Notes:

Notes:

Notes:

Notes: